KATE HALE

Developmental Delays and Interventions

Recognizing Signs and Taking Action Early

Contents

Introduction

U nderstanding Developmental Delays

Developmental delays are a common concern for many parents and caregivers, especially when a child is not meeting the typical milestones expected for their age. Developmental delays can occur in various areas, including physical, cognitive, language, and social-emotional development. It is crucial to understand these delays, their impact, and why early recognition and intervention are important. This chapter delves into the concept of developmental delays, their significance, and the misconceptions that surround them.

The Importance of Early Recognition

One of the most critical aspects of dealing with developmental delays is early recognition. Identifying developmental delays at an early stage can significantly improve a child's long-term outcomes. The early years of a child's life, particularly the first three years, represent a period of rapid growth and development. During this time, the brain is highly plastic, meaning that it can change and adapt more readily. Early intervention during this crucial period can help stimulate brain development and potentially mitigate or even resolve the effects of the delay.

Many studies show that children who receive early intervention services are more likely to reach their full potential in terms of speech, mobility, cognition, and emotional development. These services provide targeted support for children with delays, helping them develop the skills they need to succeed in school and in life. Early recognition and intervention can also help alleviate the emotional burden on parents and caregivers, as they are able to access the resources and support needed to help their child.

Additionally, recognizing developmental delays early gives parents and professionals the opportunity to monitor a child's progress over time. This can help determine whether the delay is a temporary variation in development or part of a larger, more persistent issue. Early detection also allows for timely referrals to specialists who can offer targeted therapies and support.

In practice, early recognition involves closely monitoring a child's growth and development, paying attention to their behavior, and knowing the typical developmental milestones for their age. Parents, caregivers, and healthcare providers should be aware of these milestones and take note if a child is not meeting them. Regular well-child visits with pediatricians often include developmental screenings that can help identify any concerns early on.

What Are Developmental Delays?

Developmental delays occur when a child does not achieve the developmental milestones expected for their age in one or more areas of functioning. These delays can affect a range of abilities, including physical movement, communication, cognition, and emotional regulation. It is important to distinguish between temporary developmental variations, which many children experience as they grow, and true developmental delays that require attention and intervention.

The main areas of development where delays can occur include:

1. Physical Development: This involves gross motor skills, such as sitting, crawling, walking, and running, as well as fine motor skills, like using utensils,

writing, or picking up small objects. A delay in physical development may be noticed if a child is significantly behind their peers in learning to walk or perform other motor tasks.

2. Cognitive Development: Cognitive development refers to a child's ability to think, learn, and solve problems. A delay in this area may manifest as difficulty with memory, attention, reasoning, or problem-solving tasks. Children with cognitive delays might struggle with tasks like recognizing shapes, sorting objects, or understanding cause and effect.

3. Language and Communication Development: Delays in language and communication skills can be identified when a child is not talking as much as other children their age, has trouble forming sentences, or struggles to understand what others are saying. This can include both expressive language (using words and gestures to communicate) and receptive language (understanding what others are saying).

4. Social and Emotional Development: Social and emotional development is crucial for building relationships, managing emotions, and interacting with others. A child with delays in this area might have difficulty with emotional regulation, interacting with peers, or forming relationships. For example, they may struggle to make eye contact, show empathy, or understand social cues.

5. Sensory Development: Some children experience delays in processing sensory information, such as touch, sound, or light. Sensory processing delays can make it difficult for a child to cope with certain environments, leading to behaviors like avoiding touch, covering ears in loud places, or becoming overly stimulated by bright lights.

While developmental delays can sometimes be isolated to one specific area, it is common for delays in one area to impact other areas of a child's development. For instance, a delay in language development can affect a child's social skills and emotional regulation, as they may struggle to communicate their needs and form relationships with peers.

Common Myths About Developmental Delays

There are several misconceptions about developmental delays that can prevent parents and caregivers from recognizing the signs or seeking help. These myths can contribute to a delay in intervention, which is why it is important to address and debunk them.

1. Myth: "Boys develop slower than girls, so there's no need to worry."

While it is true that there can be some gender differences in the pace of development, such as boys tending to develop language skills slightly later than girls, significant delays should not be dismissed based on gender alone. Both boys and girls are expected to reach certain milestones by specific ages, and any significant lag in reaching these milestones should be addressed.

2. Myth: "The child will grow out of it."

One of the most pervasive myths is that children will naturally "catch up" and outgrow developmental delays without intervention. While some children may outgrow minor delays or temporary developmental variations, more significant delays often require professional help. Ignoring delays in the hope that a child will outgrow them can result in missed opportunities for early intervention, which can have long-lasting effects on a child's ability to thrive.

3. Myth: "Parents did something wrong to cause the delay."

Many parents feel guilt or shame when their child is diagnosed with a developmental delay, believing that their parenting is to blame. In reality, most developmental delays are caused by a complex interplay of genetic, biological, and environmental factors. While certain environmental influences, such as prenatal exposure to alcohol or drugs, can contribute to developmental delays, parents are not typically the direct cause of their child's challenges. Rather than focusing on blame, it is more productive to concentrate on the actions that can be taken to support the child's development.

4. Myth: "Developmental delays are always permanent."

Developmental delays are not always permanent. With early and appropriate intervention, many children can overcome delays or make significant progress. The degree of improvement depends on the nature of the delay, the timing of the intervention, and the child's unique circumstances. While some delays, particularly those related to genetic or neurological conditions, may be more persistent, many children with developmental delays can lead fulfilling and independent lives with the right support.

5. Myth: "Only children from disadvantaged backgrounds experience developmental delays."

Developmental delays can occur in children from all backgrounds, regardless of sociology-economic status. While certain risk factors, such as poor prenatal care or limited access to healthcare, can increase the likelihood of developmental delays, they are not exclusive to children from disadvantaged environments. Genetic factors, birth complications, and other influences can contribute to developmental delays in children from a wide range of backgrounds.

6. Myth: "If a child has a developmental delay, they cannot succeed academically."

Having a developmental delay does not preclude a child from succeeding in school or other areas of life. Many children with delays, particularly those who receive early and targeted intervention, go on to perform well academically and socially. In many cases, tailored education plans and support services help children with developmental delays thrive in the classroom. With the right accommodations, children can overcome barriers to learning and achieve success.

7. Myth: "Developmental delays are always linked to intellectual disabilities."

Developmental delays are not synonymous with intellectual disabilities. While some children with developmental delays may also have intellectual disabilities, the two are distinct conditions. A child can have a developmental delay in one or more areas, such as language or motor skills, without having a global intellectual disability. It is important to assess each child's unique strengths and challenges individually, rather than making assumptions based on a delay in one area of development.

Final Thought

Understanding the nature of developmental delays, their causes, and the importance of early intervention is crucial for parents, caregivers, and professionals. By recognizing the signs early, seeking appropriate assessments, and accessing resources, children with developmental delays can receive the support they need to reach their full potential. Dispelling the myths surrounding developmental delays is equally important, as it helps parents approach the situation with clarity, confidence, and a proactive mindset. Recognizing that early intervention can make a significant difference encourages timely action, ensuring that children receive the best possible start in life.

Milestones in Child Development

C hild development is a dynamic and multifaceted process that involves the acquisition of various skills across physical, cognitive, and emotional domains. Each child grows at their own pace, but there are universal milestones that serve as general benchmarks for what most children achieve by a certain age. These milestones are crucial indicators of a child's developmental progress and provide insights into typical versus atypical development. Understanding these milestones helps parents, caregivers, and professionals monitor a child's growth and identify any delays early on, allowing for timely intervention and support when necessary.

Physical, Cognitive, and Emotional Milestones

Child development can be broken down into several domains, with each playing a critical role in a child's overall growth and ability to interact with the world. The three major domains of development include physical, cognitive, and emotional milestones.

Physical Milestones refer to the development of both gross and fine motor skills. Gross motor skills involve large movements like crawling, walking, running, and jumping, whereas fine motor skills involve smaller, more precise movements such as grasping objects, drawing, or using utensils. A child's ability to gain physical control over their body is an essential part of their development, enabling them to explore their environment, gain independence, and perform daily tasks.

For instance, in infancy, physical milestones include head control, rolling over, sitting up, and crawling. By the toddler years, children typically walk, run, and climb. As preschoolers, they refine their physical abilities further by learning to hop, balance on one foot, ride a tricycle, and use scissors or draw simple shapes. Fine motor skills become increasingly important as children prepare for school, learning to write their names, manipulate small objects, and complete tasks that require dexterity.

Cognitive Milestones involve the development of intellectual abilities such as thinking, problem-solving, memory, and understanding cause-and-effect relationships. These milestones are critical for how children learn, adapt to new situations, and make sense of the world around them. Cognitive development enables children to process information, build knowledge, and develop skills that form the foundation for more complex learning later in life.

Early cognitive milestones include the ability to recognize familiar faces, track moving objects, and explore through touch and taste. As children grow, they develop more advanced cognitive abilities like following simple directions, solving puzzles, and recognizing shapes, colors, and numbers. By preschool age, children begin to understand time, cause and effect, and are able to engage in imaginative play, an important aspect of cognitive development that involves abstract thinking and creativity.

Emotional Milestones are concerned with the development of self-awareness, emotional regulation, and social interaction. Emotional development is critical for forming healthy relationships, managing emotions, and navigating social situations. Children who develop strong emotional skills are better equipped to handle challenges, express themselves, and engage positively with others.

In infancy, emotional milestones include forming attachments with caregivers, expressing basic emotions like happiness, sadness, and anger, and beginning to recognize familiar faces. Toddlers develop a sense of autonomy and begin to assert independence, often resulting in temper tantrums as they navigate strong emotions like frustration and excitement. By preschool age, children start to understand and manage their emotions better, display empathy, and develop friendships. They also learn to follow rules, share with peers, and resolve conflicts with guidance.

When to Expect Key Milestones (0–5 Years)

The first five years of life are critical for a child's development, with each year marking significant progress in physical, cognitive, and emotional milestones. Below is an overview of when to expect key milestones during this period.

0–6 Months: In the first six months of life, infants undergo rapid growth and development, particularly in the areas of physical and sensory skills. At this stage, babies typically gain control of their head, start reaching for objects, and respond to stimuli such as sounds, lights, and faces. Cognitive development during this period includes recognizing familiar voices, reacting to their name, and showing interest in their surroundings. Emotionally, infants form strong bonds with their primary caregivers, displaying attachment behaviors like smiling and crying for attention.

- Physical Milestones: Lifting head, rolling over, grasping objects.
  - Cognitive Milestones: Recognizing familiar faces, following moving objects with eyes.
  - Emotional Milestones: Smiling in response to attention, forming attachment to caregivers.

6–12 Months: Between six months and one year, babies become more mobile, learning to sit up, crawl, and eventually take their first steps. They also begin to develop fine motor skills, such as picking up small objects using a pincer grasp. Cognitively, infants start to understand simple instructions, like "no" or "come here," and demonstrate curiosity by exploring their environment. Emotionally, they may show separation anxiety when away from caregivers and begin to exhibit a wider range of emotions.

- Physical Milestones: Sitting up without support, crawling, pulling to stand, and possibly walking.
  - Cognitive Milestones: Responding to name, understanding basic instructions, exploring objects.
  - Emotional Milestones: Separation anxiety, showing a range of emotions such as joy and frustration.

1–2 Years: The toddler years bring significant advances in all areas of development. Physically, most toddlers walk independently, run, and begin to climb. Fine motor skills continue to develop as they learn to feed themselves, stack blocks, and scribble with crayons. Cognitive development includes the ability to solve simple problems, follow two-step instructions, and name objects or people. Emotionally, toddlers assert their independence, leading to behaviors like temper tantrums when they are frustrated or unable to communicate their needs.

- Physical Milestones: Walking, running, climbing, feeding themselves.
  - Cognitive Milestones: Identifying objects, following simple instructions, solving basic problems.
  - Emotional Milestones: Developing independence, experiencing strong emotions, temper tantrums.

2–3 Years: Between ages two and three, children refine their gross and fine motor skills, improving their coordination and control. They become more proficient at activities like jumping, throwing, and catching, as well as using utensils and drawing simple shapes. Cognitive development includes understanding the concept of "mine" and "yours," recognizing colors, and engaging in pretend play. Emotionally, children become more aware of their own feelings and the feelings of others, often displaying empathy and starting to develop friendships.

- Physical Milestones: Jumping, running more steadily, using utensils, drawing simple shapes.
  - Cognitive Milestones: Recognizing colors, engaging in imaginative play, understanding simple concepts like ownership.
  - Emotional Milestones: Showing empathy, beginning to make friends, managing emotions with guidance.

3–4 Years: At this stage, children become more independent and capable in terms of physical tasks. They can ride a tricycle, dress themselves with minimal help, and use scissors to cut paper. Cognitive abilities continue to expand, as they understand time (e.g., "yesterday" and "tomorrow"), count to ten, and use sentences to express ideas clearly. Emotional development includes greater emotional regulation, cooperation with peers, and the ability to share and take turns during play.

- Physical Milestones: Riding a tricycle, dressing themselves, using scissors.
  - Cognitive Milestones: Counting to ten, understanding time concepts, forming longer sentences.
  - Emotional Milestones: Improved emotional regulation, sharing with others, building friendships.

4–5 Years: By the time a child reaches four to five years of age, they are typically able to perform more complex physical tasks, such as hopping on one foot, catching a ball reliably, and writing some letters. Cognitive development includes the ability to understand and follow more complex instructions, identify numbers and letters, and engage in more structured play that follows rules. Emotionally, children at this age develop a stronger sense of identity, build deeper relationships with peers, and show an increased capacity for empathy and cooperation.

- Physical Milestones: Hopping on one foot, catching a ball, writing some letters.
  - Cognitive Milestones: Identifying letters and numbers, following multi-step instructions, engaging in structured play.
  - Emotional Milestones: Stronger sense of identity, forming deeper friendships, displaying cooperation and empathy.

Typical vs. Atypical Development

While there are general timelines for when children are expected to achieve certain developmental milestones, it is important to understand that every child develops at their own pace. Some children may reach milestones earlier than expected, while others may take a little longer to catch up. Variations in the timing of milestones are typically normal and are not always a cause for concern. However, it is also essential to be aware of the difference between typical and atypical development, as delays in meeting key milestones can sometimes signal an underlying issue.

Typical Development refers to the general progression of skills that most children acquire within a certain age range. For example, most children will start walking between 9 and 15 months, say their first words around 12 months, and engage in pretend play by the age of 2. Typical development follows a relatively predictable pattern, although the exact timing of milestone achievement can vary from child to child.

Parents and caregivers should keep in mind that temporary delays in development do not necessarily indicate a problem. For instance, some children may be early walkers but late talkers, or vice versa. The focus should be on the overall trajectory of the child's development rather than a strict adherence to specific timelines.

Atypical Development, on the other hand, refers to significant deviations from the expected range of milestones. Children with atypical development may show delays in one or more areas of development, such as motor skills, language, or emotional regulation. For example, a child who is not walking by 18 months or not speaking any words by 2 years old may be exhibiting signs of atypical development, which could warrant further assessment or intervention.

One of the key indicators of atypical development is when a child consistently misses multiple milestones in one or more areas of development, especially if they show little to no progress over time. It's important to note that developmental delays are not always indicative of a long-term or permanent issue; some children simply develop at a slower pace but eventually catch up. However, when delays are persistent, or when they are accompanied by other concerning behaviors (such as a lack of interest in interaction or repetitive, restricted behaviors), it may be a sign of a developmental disorder, such as autism spectrum disorder (ASD), cerebral palsy, or intellectual disability.

In assessing whether a child's development is typical or atypical, healthcare professionals use various screening tools and assessments to measure a child's performance in relation to expected milestones. These assessments are designed to take into account the wide range of normal variation in child development while identifying red flags that could signal a need for further evaluation.

Red Flags for Atypical Development by Age

- By 6 Months: Lack of eye contact, minimal interest in engaging with caregivers, difficulty holding head up, not rolling over.
  - By 12 Months: No babbling, not responding to name, not sitting up without support, lack of interest in exploring surroundings.
  - By 18 Months: No walking, no use of single words, inability to point to show interest, limited social interaction.
  - By 24 Months: No two-word phrases, difficulty with coordination or walking, inability to follow simple instructions, little to no interest in playing

with other children.

- By 3 Years: Difficulty speaking in short sentences, limited vocabulary, trouble with motor tasks like jumping or climbing, inability to engage in imaginative play.

- By 4–5 Years: Difficulty recognizing basic concepts like colors or shapes, inability to follow multi-step directions, poor coordination, inability to form friendships or follow group activities.

While some children may experience delays in one or two areas, these red flags often signal that further assessment may be needed. Delays in reaching milestones could be due to a variety of factors, including genetic conditions, neurological disorders, environmental influences, or sensory processing difficulties. Therefore, when children miss several key milestones or exhibit developmental patterns that differ significantly from their peers, it is essential to consult with a healthcare provider to determine the underlying cause and create a plan for early intervention.

Factors That Influence Development

Several factors can affect whether a child reaches developmental milestones on time or experiences delays. Some of these factors are biological, while others are environmental or situational. Understanding these influences can provide valuable context when evaluating a child's developmental progress.

1. Genetics: A child's genetic makeup plays a significant role in their developmental trajectory. Certain conditions, such as Down syndrome or Fragile X syndrome, are directly linked to genetic variations that affect cognitive, physical, and emotional development. In some cases, family history of developmental delays may also indicate an increased likelihood of delays in children.

2. Premature and Birth Complications: Babies born prematurely may take longer to reach certain milestones compared to full-term infants.

Developmental delays are more common in premature infants because their organs and nervous systems are less developed at birth. Complications during birth, such as oxygen deprivation or traumatic delivery, can also impact a child's developmental progress.

3. Prenatal Environment: A mother's health during pregnancy can influence a child's development. Factors like maternal nutrition, exposure to toxins (such as alcohol, tobacco, or drugs), and stress levels during pregnancy can all contribute to developmental outcomes. Prenatal care and proper management of maternal health conditions (such as gestational diabetes or hypertension) are important in reducing the risk of developmental delays.

4. Postnatal Environment: After birth, a child's environment continues to shape their development. Children raised in stimulating, nurturing environments are more likely to reach developmental milestones on time. In contrast, neglect, abuse, or lack of access to enriching activities can contribute to developmental delays. Children from lower sociology-economic backgrounds may face additional challenges due to limited access to healthcare, early education, and other developmental resources.

5. Health and Nutrition: Proper nutrition during the early years is essential for brain development and physical growth. Deficiencies in key nutrients (such as iron, iodine, or omega-3 fatty acids) can negatively affect cognitive and motor development. Additionally, chronic health conditions, infections, or frequent illnesses can interfere with a child's ability to meet milestones.

6. Parental Involvement: The level of interaction a child has with caregivers also impacts their development. Parents who engage their children through play, reading, and conversation help foster cognitive, social, and emotional skills. On the other hand, children who receive minimal interaction or stimulation may struggle to reach certain milestones, particularly in the areas of language and social development.

The Importance of Regular Monitoring and Checkups

Regular developmental screenings and well-child checkups are critical in identifying potential developmental delays. Pediatricians typically assess a child's growth and progress at regular intervals, particularly during the first few years of life, when development is most rapid. These screenings involve observing the child's behavior, asking parents about developmental milestones, and sometimes using standardized tools to measure the child's performance.

For parents, it's important to attend all scheduled well-child visits and communicate any concerns they may have about their child's development. Developmental delays may not always be obvious, especially in children who show uneven patterns of growth (e.g., a child who excels in physical development but lags in language). Parents and caregivers should remain vigilant, as they are often the first to notice subtle signs that something may be amiss. If a delay is suspected, the pediatrician may refer the child to a specialist for further evaluation, such as a speech therapist, occupational therapist, or developmental psychologist.

Intervention and Support for Developmental Delays

Early intervention is key to helping children with developmental delays reach their full potential. Research consistently shows that the earlier a child receives help, the better their outcomes in terms of academic achievement, social skills, and overall well-being. In the United States, early intervention programs are available to children from birth to age three through the Individuals with Disabilities Education Act (IDEA) Part C. These services are designed to provide individualized support for children with developmental delays, focusing on areas such as speech therapy, occupational therapy, physical therapy, and behavioral support.

Once a child is identified as having a delay, professionals work with the family to create an Individualized Family Service Plan (IFSP), which outlines specific goals and interventions tailored to the child's needs. Early intervention services are usually provided in the child's home or in a community setting, making it easier for parents to be involved in the process. The goal is to support the child's development through play-based activities and structured learning that can be integrated into daily routines.

As children grow older, if delays persist, they may transition to special education services through public school systems. School-based interventions are governed by IDEA Part B, which provides for an Individualized Education Plan (IEP) for children aged three to twenty-one. These services may include specialized instruction, classroom accommodations, and access to therapists who work on specific developmental goals. The ultimate aim of these programs is to help children participate fully in the academic environment and reach their developmental potential.

The Role of Parents and Caregivers in Supporting Development

Parents and caregivers play a vital role in supporting a child's development, both in terms of preventing delays and addressing them when they arise. Engaging in age-appropriate activities that stimulate a child's physical, cognitive, and emotional growth can make a significant difference in their ability to reach milestones. Activities such as reading to a child, engaging in conversation, providing opportunities for physical play, and encouraging problem-solving all contribute to well-rounded development.

Additionally, parents should remain informed about typical child development and familiarize themselves with the milestones children are expected to reach. Resources such as developmental milestone checklists, parenting guides, and consultations with healthcare providers can help parents track their child's progress and identify potential concerns. When a delay is suspected, early intervention programs often include training for parents so they can continue supporting their child's growth at home.

In some cases, managing a child with developmental delays can be challenging, particularly if the child has additional needs or behaviors that require ongoing attention. It is important for parents to seek out support networks, including local early intervention services, parent advocacy groups, and online communities where they can share experiences and obtain guidance.

: Milestones as a Guide, Not a Rigid Timeline

Developmental milestones are a valuable tool for understanding and monitoring a child's progress. However, they should be seen as general guidelines rather than rigid timelines that every child must follow precisely. Children develop at different rates, and some variation is normal. That said, when children consistently miss key milestones, it is important to address the issue with appropriate screenings and interventions to ensure that they receive the support they need to thrive.

The early years of life are full of rapid changes, and each child's developmental journey is unique. By staying informed, being proactive about potential concerns, and embracing early intervention when necessary, parents and caregivers can give their children the best possible start. Regular monitoring, a supportive environment, and targeted intervention can help children with developmental delays reach their potential and overcome challenges along the way.

Recognizing the Signs of Developmental Delays

Recognizing the early signs of developmental delays is critical in providing timely intervention and support to children. Developmental delays can manifest in various forms, affecting a child's ability to communicate, move, interact socially, or process sensory information. These delays are often categorized into different domains, including speech and language, motor skills, social and emotional development, cognitive development, and sensory processing. Each area of development plays a key role in a child's overall growth and ability to function in daily life. By understanding the specific signs of delays in each domain, parents, caregivers, and educators can better identify potential concerns and seek appropriate help.

Speech and Language Delays

Speech and language development is a critical aspect of early childhood growth, as it underpins communication and social interaction. Delays in this area can significantly impact a child's ability to express themselves, understand others, and engage in meaningful conversations. Speech and language delays are among the most common developmental delays, and they can present in several ways, including delayed speech, difficulty understanding language, or challenges in forming coherent sentences.

Delayed Speech is one of the earliest signs that parents may notice. Children typically begin to babble by around six months, say their first words by twelve months, and combine words into simple phrases by the age of two. If a child is not meeting these milestones, it could be a sign of a speech delay. For example, a child who is not saying any words by eighteen months or who is not forming two-word phrases by age two may have a speech delay. Children with speech delays may also struggle with pronunciation, making it difficult for others to understand them.

Language comprehension issues are another sign of a potential delay. While speech refers to the ability to articulate sounds and words, language encompasses the understanding and use of words and sentences. A child with a language delay may have trouble following simple instructions, answering questions, or recognizing familiar words. For instance, if a two-year-old does not understand basic commands like "come here" or "give me the toy," this could indicate a receptive language delay. In some cases, children with language delays can speak but have difficulty making sense of what others are saying, which can lead to frustration and behavioral issues.

Children with expressive language delays may understand what is being said but have difficulty putting their thoughts into words. These children might use gestures or sounds to communicate instead of words, or they may rely on short, incomplete sentences that lack grammatical structure. For example, a three-year-old who should be able to form sentences might instead use single words or point to objects rather than naming them. Expressive language delays can affect a child's ability to participate in conversations, make requests, or share their thoughts.

In some cases, speech and language delays may be associated with other conditions, such as autism spectrum disorder (ASD) or hearing impairments. Hearing problems, for example, can cause delays in speech because the child is not receiving the auditory input needed to learn how to speak. Children with autism may also experience delays in language development, particularly in the area of social communication, such as understanding nonverbal cues or taking turns in conversation.

Warning signs of speech and language delays include:
   - By 6 months: Lack of babbling or cooing, not responding to sounds.
   - By 12 months: Not saying single words, not using gestures like waving or pointing.
   - By 18 months: Limited vocabulary, difficulty understanding simple commands.
   - By 24 months: Not forming two-word phrases, not recognizing familiar words or objects.
   - By 3 years: Difficulty with pronunciation, inability to form simple sentences, lack of interest in social interactions through speech.

Motor Skill Delays

Motor skills encompass both gross motor skills (large movements involving the whole body, like crawling, walking, and running) and fine motor skills (small movements involving the hands and fingers, like grasping, drawing, or using utensils). Delays in motor skill development can affect a child's ability to explore their environment, perform everyday tasks, and engage in play. These delays can be caused by a variety of factors, including genetic conditions, neurological disorders, or environmental influences.

Gross motor delays refer to difficulties with large muscle movements. Children typically develop gross motor skills in a predictable sequence, starting with head control, rolling over, sitting up, crawling, standing, and eventually walking and running. A child who does not meet these milestones within the expected time frame may have a gross motor delay. For example, a baby who is not sitting up by nine months or not walking by eighteen months may be experiencing a delay in gross motor development.

In some cases, children with gross motor delays may appear clumsy or uncoordinated. They might struggle with balance, have difficulty running or climbing, or avoid activities that require physical exertion. These children may also have poor posture, tire easily during physical activities, or prefer to remain sedentary. Gross motor delays can affect a child's ability to participate in sports, playground activities, or even basic self-care tasks like dressing or bathing.

Fine motor delays involve difficulty with smaller, more precise movements, such as grasping objects, using utensils, or drawing. Fine motor skills are important for tasks like writing, cutting with scissors, and manipulating small objects. A child with fine motor delays may have trouble holding a pencil, stacking blocks, or using buttons and zippers. For example, a three-year-old who cannot draw a simple circle or a four-year-old who struggles to hold a crayon properly may be exhibiting signs of a fine motor delay.

Fine motor delays can also impact a child's ability to perform self-care tasks, such as feeding themselves, brushing their teeth, or tying their shoes. These delays can lead to frustration and a lack of independence, as the child may rely on caregivers for tasks that their peers can perform on their own.

Warning signs of motor skill delays include:
   - By 6 months: Not rolling over, difficulty lifting head, lack of interest in reaching for objects.
   - By 12 months: Not sitting up independently, not crawling, not standing with support.
   - By 18 months: Not walking, difficulty with balance or coordination, not using hands to explore objects.
   - By 2 years: Not running, climbing, or kicking a ball, difficulty with hand-eye coordination.
   - By 3 years: Not drawing simple shapes, difficulty using utensils, trouble dressing themselves.

Social and Emotional Delays

Social and emotional development is essential for building relationships, managing emotions, and navigating social situations. Delays in this area can affect a child's ability to interact with others, regulate their emotions, and form meaningful connections with peers and caregivers. Social and emotional delays are often associated with developmental disorders such as autism spectrum disorder (ASD), attention deficit hyperactivity disorder (ADHD), or anxiety disorders.

Social delays refer to difficulties with interacting with others, understanding social cues, and engaging in reciprocal communication. Children typically begin to develop social skills in infancy, such as smiling in response to caregivers, making eye contact, and engaging in back-and-forth interactions. A child with a social delay may avoid eye contact, prefer to play alone, or have difficulty understanding the emotions of others. For example, a toddler who does not engage in pretend play, avoids group activities, or does not show interest in interacting with peers may be exhibiting signs of a social delay.

As children grow, social delays can impact their ability to make friends, follow rules, and participate in group activities. A preschooler with social delays may struggle to take turns, share with others, or follow simple social rules, such as waiting in line or listening to a teacher. These challenges can lead to social isolation, frustration, and difficulty adapting to school environments.

Emotional delays involve difficulties with emotional regulation, understanding feelings, and responding appropriately to emotions. Children typically learn to identify and express their emotions in healthy ways, such as using words to describe how they feel or seeking comfort from caregivers when upset. A child with emotional delays may have frequent temper tantrums, become easily overwhelmed by strong emotions, or have trouble calming down after being upset.

For instance, a child who consistently has meltdowns when transitioning from one activity to another or who is unable to soothe themselves when distressed may be exhibiting signs of an emotional delay. Emotional delays can also manifest as difficulty showing empathy or understanding the feelings of others, leading to challenges in forming relationships with peers and caregivers.

Warning signs of social and emotional delays include:
- By 6 months: Lack of smiling or eye contact, limited interest in interacting with caregivers.
- By 12 months: Not responding to name, not engaging in back-and-forth interactions, not showing interest in social games like peek-a-boo.
- By 2 years: Preferring to play alone, difficulty taking turns, lack of pretend play.
- By 3 years: Difficulty regulating emotions, frequent temper tantrums, inability to form friendships.
- By 4–5 years: Struggling with group activities, inability to express emotions in appropriate ways, difficulty understanding social rules.

Cognitive Delays

Cognitive development refers to a child's ability to think, learn, and solve problems. Cognitive delays can affect a child's ability to process information, understand cause-and-effect relationships, and engage in higher-order thinking. Children with cognitive delays may struggle with memory, attention, reasoning, and problem-solving skills, which can impact their academic performance and ability to engage in everyday tasks.

Cognitive delays may present in infancy, with a child showing little curiosity about their environment or difficulty learning new skills. For example, a baby who does not respond to stimuli like lights or sounds or who shows little interest in exploring objects may be exhibiting signs of a cognitive delay. As children grow older, cognitive delays may become more apparent in areas like language development, problem-solving, and understanding basic concepts.

Children with cognitive delays may have difficulty following instructions, completing puzzles, or understanding abstract concepts like time or numbers. For example, a preschool-aged child who struggles to count, recognize shapes, or follow multi-step instructions may be showing signs of a cognitive delay. These delays can affect not only academic abilities but also everyday problem-solving skills, such as figuring out how to complete a task or solve a basic puzzle.

Cognitive delays can vary in severity. Some children may show mild difficulties that become apparent only when they reach school age, while others may experience more significant challenges early on. Children with cognitive delays may also struggle with executive functioning skills, such as planning, organizing, and regulating attention. This can make it difficult for them to manage tasks that require focus and sustained effort.

It's also important to note that cognitive delays are sometimes associated with other developmental issues, such as learning disabilities, intellectual disabilities, or developmental disorders like autism spectrum disorder (ASD). Children with cognitive delays may need individualized educational plans (IEPs) or specialized interventions to support their learning and help them reach their full potential.

Warning signs of cognitive delays include:
- By 6 months: Limited curiosity, not exploring objects, difficulty tracking objects visually.
- By 12 months: Not recognizing familiar people or objects, not understanding simple words or gestures.
- By 18 months: Not following simple instructions, difficulty with cause-and-effect toys, limited problem-solving abilities.
- By 2 years: Not recognizing basic concepts like size or shape, inability to follow two-step directions.
- By 3 years: Difficulty with memory, attention, and understanding abstract concepts like numbers or time.

Sensory Processing Issues

Sensory processing refers to how the brain interprets and responds to information received from the senses, such as sight, sound, touch, taste, and smell. Some children have difficulty processing sensory input, which can lead to sensory processing issues. These issues can manifest as either hypersensitivity (over-responsiveness) or hypo-sensitivity (under-responsiveness) to sensory stimuli. Children with sensory processing issues may struggle to integrate sensory information in a way that allows them to function comfortably in their environment.

Children with hypersensitivity may be easily overwhelmed by everyday sensory experiences. For example, they might cover their ears in response to loud noises, become distressed by bright lights, or refuse to wear certain fabrics because they feel uncomfortable. Hypersensitive children may also have difficulty with food textures, avoiding certain foods or gagging when presented with unfamiliar textures. These children are often described as "sensitive" or "picky" because they react strongly to stimuli that others might not notice.

On the other hand, children with hypo-sensitivity may seek out sensory input or seem unresponsive to stimuli that others find uncomfortable. For example, they might not react to pain, fail to notice loud sounds, or crave intense sensory experiences like spinning or swinging. These children may engage in repetitive behaviors like rocking or spinning to self-regulate, or they may seek out rough physical play. Hypo-sensitive children may also have delayed responses to sensory input, such as not reacting to being touched or not noticing when they are dirty or wet.

Sensory processing issues can affect many areas of a child's development, including motor skills, behavior, and social interaction. For example, a child who is hypersensitive to sound may have trouble participating in group activities at school, while a child with hypo-sensitivity may have difficulty recognizing physical boundaries during play. Sensory issues can also lead to challenges with self-regulation, making it hard for children to calm down when overstimulated or focus when under-stimulated.

Children with sensory processing issues may benefit from occupational therapy, which helps them develop strategies for managing sensory input and improving their ability to function in daily life. Occupational therapists often use sensory integration therapy, which involves structured activities designed to help the child gradually adapt to different sensory experiences.

Warning signs of sensory processing issues include:
- By 6 months: Overly sensitive to lights, sounds, or textures, or not reacting to sensory stimuli at all.
- By 12 months: Strong aversion to certain textures, sounds, or lights, or constantly seeking out sensory input through movement or touch.
- By 18 months: Difficulty calming down after being overstimulated, or showing little to no reaction to loud noises or touch.
- By 2 years: Avoidance of certain sensory experiences, such as specific foods or textures, or excessive seeking of sensory input.
- By 3 years: Difficulty participating in group activities due to sensory sensitivities, or engaging in repetitive sensory-seeking behaviors like spinning or rocking.

Recognizing the signs of developmental delays in speech and language, motor skills, social and emotional development, cognitive abilities, and sensory processing is crucial for ensuring that children receive the support they need to reach their full potential. Early detection and intervention are key to addressing developmental challenges and helping children thrive in their everyday lives. By being vigilant and responsive to potential delays, parents, caregivers, and educators can play an essential role in supporting children's growth and development.

Diagnosing Developmental Delays

D evelopmental delays can manifest in various ways across cognitive, physical, emotional, and social domains. Identifying these delays early on is essential for ensuring timely intervention and support, which can drastically improve outcomes for children. Diagnosis is a multi-step process that involves various professionals, tools, and assessments to determine whether a child is meeting the expected developmental milestones for their age. This chapter will explore the role of pediatricians and early screenings, the various developmental screening tools and assessments used in diagnosing developmental delays, and how parents and caregivers can best prepare for a formal diagnosis.

The Role of Pediatricians and Early Screenings

Pediatricians play a critical role in identifying potential developmental delays. Routine visits to the pediatrician, especially in the first few years of a child's life, are designed not only to monitor physical health but also to assess developmental progress. These well-child visits are pivotal in the early detection of developmental issues, as pediatricians are trained to observe a wide range of behaviors and developmental markers.

During regular checkups, pediatricians perform developmental surveillance, which involves tracking a child's developmental progress over time. They may ask parents about their child's behavior, interaction with others, and progress toward reaching developmental milestones. These conversations provide valuable insight into the child's growth, as parents are often the first to notice subtle changes or delays in their child's development.

Pediatricians often rely on their clinical judgment, combined with input from parents, to assess whether a child's development is progressing typically or if there are areas of concern. They use established developmental milestones, which include age-appropriate expectations for physical, cognitive, social, and language skills, as benchmarks. For example, at a 12-month visit, a pediatrician will check if the child is crawling, babbling, and responding to their name. At 24 months, they may observe whether the child is using two-word phrases, walking confidently, and showing interest in playing with others.

In addition to these informal observations, pediatricians use standardized screening tools at key developmental stages to gather more structured data on a child's abilities. The American Academy of Pediatrics (AAP) recommends that pediatricians conduct formal developmental screenings at specific intervals, particularly at 9, 18, and 24 or 30 months. These screenings help detect any deviations from typical developmental patterns and provide a basis for further evaluation.

For children who show signs of developmental delays, pediatricians act as gatekeepers, coordinating further evaluations and referrals to specialists. Depending on the child's needs, this may involve referring the family to developmental pediatricians, neurologists, speech therapists, occupational therapists, or psychologists. Pediatricians also play an important role in guiding families through the process of seeking early intervention services, which are critical for addressing developmental delays as early as possible.

Early screenings are designed to catch delays before they become more pronounced, which is why they are often performed at regular intervals during a child's first few years. These screenings are especially important because some developmental delays, such as speech and language delays or cognitive delays, may not be immediately apparent in infancy but become more obvious as the child reaches preschool age. Early identification allows for the prompt initiation of interventions, which can significantly improve outcomes for children with developmental delays.

Parents also play a key role in this process by providing accurate and detailed information about their child's behavior and progress. Pediatricians often rely on parental observations, as children may not exhibit certain behaviors during short office visits. Parents are encouraged to speak up about any concerns they have regarding their child's development, even if these concerns seem minor, as early intervention can prevent small delays from becoming larger issues.

Developmental Screening Tools and Assessments

Developmental screenings and assessments are crucial components of the diagnostic process for identifying developmental delays. These tools are designed to measure a child's abilities across different domains, including motor skills, language, cognitive development, and social-emotional functioning. Screening tools are typically used to identify children who may be at risk for delays and require further evaluation, while assessments provide a more in-depth analysis of a child's strengths and challenges.

Screening Tools: Developmental screening tools are standardized instruments used by healthcare professionals, educators, and sometimes parents to quickly assess a child's progress toward developmental milestones. These tools are often questionnaires or checklists that are easy to administer and interpret. They help determine whether a child is developing typically or if there may be a need for further evaluation. Some of the most commonly used screening tools include:

1. Ages and Stages Questionnaire (ASQ): The ASQ is one of the most widely used screening tools for young children. It covers five developmental

domains: communication, gross motor skills, fine motor skills, problem-solving, and personal-social skills. The ASQ is completed by parents, which allows them to provide information about their child's behavior and abilities in the home environment. The questionnaire is designed to be easy to understand and can be administered at multiple stages, from infancy through preschool age.

2. Pediatric Evaluation of Developmental Status (PEDS): The PEDS is a brief questionnaire that helps identify developmental and behavioral problems in children. It asks parents to report on any concerns they have about their child's development, behavior, and learning. The PEDS is often used in conjunction with other screening tools to provide a more comprehensive picture of the child's developmental status.

3. Modified Checklist for Autism in Toddlers (M-CHAT): The M-CHAT is a screening tool specifically designed to identify children who may be at risk for autism spectrum disorder (ASD). It is typically administered between 16 and 30 months of age. The M-CHAT includes questions about social communication, eye contact, and play behaviors, which are key areas of concern for children with ASD.

4. Denver Developmental Screening Test (DDST): The DDST assesses a child's performance in four key areas: personal-social, fine motor-adaptive, language, and gross motor skills. It is often used for children from birth to six years old and helps identify children who may have developmental delays.

5. Brigance Early Childhood Screens: The Brigance screens assess various aspects of development, including language, motor skills, cognitive development, and social-emotional functioning. It is commonly used in early childhood education settings and pediatric practices to screen for developmental delays and learning disabilities.

Once a child has been identified as being at risk for developmental de-

31

lays through a screening tool, the next step is a more comprehensive developmental assessment. Developmental assessments are conducted by trained professionals, such as developmental pediatricians, psychologists, or therapists, and provide a detailed analysis of a child's abilities in specific areas. These assessments are typically more time-intensive than screenings and may involve direct observation, standardized testing, and interviews with parents.

Developmental Assessments: The goal of a developmental assessment is to identify the specific areas in which a child is experiencing delays and to determine the severity of those delays. The results of these assessments help guide intervention planning and the development of individualized education or therapy plans. Some commonly used developmental assessments include:

1. Bayley Scales of Infant and Toddler Development (Bayley-III): The Bayley-III is a comprehensive assessment tool that measures a child's development across five domains: cognitive, language, motor, social-emotional, and adaptive behavior. It is often used with children from one month to 42 months old and provides a detailed picture of the child's strengths and challenges in each area. The Bayley-III is administered by a trained professional and involves direct interaction with the child, as well as questionnaires completed by parents.

2. Wechsler Preschool and Primary Scale of Intelligence (WPPSI): The WPPSI is an intelligence test designed for children between the ages of 2.5 and 7 years. It assesses cognitive abilities, including verbal comprehension, visual-spatial reasoning, working memory, and processing speed. While not specifically a developmental test, the WPPSI can provide valuable information about a child's cognitive abilities and help identify areas of concern.

3. Peabody Developmental Motor Scales (PDMS-2): The PDMS-2 assesses motor skills in children from birth to 5 years old. It evaluates both gross and fine motor abilities, including locomotion, object manipulation, grasping, and visual-motor integration. This assessment is often used by occupational

and physical therapists to identify motor skill delays and develop intervention plans.

4. Clinical Evaluation of Language Fundamentals (CELF): The CELF is a standardized assessment used to evaluate language skills in children. It measures both receptive and expressive language abilities, including vocabulary, sentence structure, and understanding of grammar. Speech therapists often use the CELF to assess children who are experiencing language delays or disorders.

5. Vineland Adaptive Behavior Scales: The Vineland scales assess adaptive behaviors, including communication, daily living skills, socialization, and motor skills. This assessment is commonly used to evaluate children with intellectual disabilities, autism spectrum disorder, and other developmental delays. The Vineland is typically completed through interviews with parents or caregivers and provides valuable information about how well the child functions in everyday life.

These assessments are critical in determining whether a child qualifies for early intervention services or special education programs. They also help professionals create individualized plans to address the child's unique needs and provide targeted support for their developmental progress.

How to Prepare for a Diagnosis

The process of diagnosing a developmental delay can be overwhelming for parents, particularly if they are unfamiliar with the terminology, procedures, and professionals involved. Preparing for a diagnosis involves gathering information, documenting concerns, and understanding the steps that will take place during the assessment. Here are some key steps for parents and caregivers to consider when preparing for a diagnosis:

1. Document Developmental Concerns: One of the most important things

parents can do is keep a detailed record of their child's behavior and development. This includes noting any delays or concerns that have arisen over time, as well as specific examples of behaviors or milestones the child has or has not reached.

Understanding the Causes of Developmental Delays

D evelopmental delays can stem from a wide variety of causes, often influenced by a combination of genetic, biological, environmental, and health-related factors. Understanding these underlying causes is critical for identifying at-risk children and implementing early interventions that can improve their outcomes. The causes of developmental delays are multifaceted, and it is important to recognize that in many cases, multiple factors may contribute to the delays. In this chapter, we will explore the major contributing causes of developmental delays, including genetic and biological factors, environmental influences, prenatal and birth complications, and the role of nutrition and early childhood health.

Genetic and Biological Factors

One of the primary causes of developmental delays is rooted in genetics and biology. Certain genetic disorders and abnormalities can significantly affect a child's development from birth and often manifest in delays across various domains, such as cognitive, motor, and social-emotional skills. In addition, biological factors like brain injuries or complications in early development can impact a child's ability to reach developmental milestones.

Genetic conditions can have a profound impact on a child's development, and many developmental delays are linked to specific genetic syndromes. Some of the most common genetic disorders that result in developmental delays include:

1. Down Syndrome: Down syndrome is a genetic condition caused by the presence of an extra copy of chromosome 21 (isometric 21). This condition is associated with intellectual disabilities, delayed speech and language development, and delayed motor skills. Children with Down syndrome may also experience slower physical growth and face challenges in social-emotional development.

2. Fragile X Syndrome: Fragile X syndrome is another genetic condition that affects brain development. It is caused by a mutation in the FMRI gene on the X chromosome. Fragile X is the most common inherited cause of intellectual disability and is often accompanied by delays in speech, language, and social skills. Children with Fragile X may also exhibit behavioral problems, such as anxiety, hyperactivity, and sensory sensitivities.

3. Rett Syndrome: Rett syndrome is a rare genetic disorder that primarily affects girls and leads to severe cognitive and motor impairments. It is caused by mutations in the MECP2 gene on the X chromosome. Children with Rett syndrome often experience normal development in the first few months of life, followed by a rapid loss of motor and communication skills. This regression is accompanied by profound developmental delays and difficulty with hand movements, balance, and coordination.

4. Autism Spectrum Disorder (ASD): Although not caused by a single genetic mutation, many cases of autism spectrum disorder are thought to have a genetic component. Research suggests that ASD may result from a combination of genetic vulnerabilities and environmental factors. Children with ASD often experience delays in social communication and may exhibit repetitive behaviors or restricted interests. These delays can vary widely in severity, with some children showing mild impairments while others face significant challenges.

5. Cerebral Palsy: Cerebral palsy is a group of neurological disorders that affect movement and coordination. It is typically caused by brain damage that occurs before, during, or shortly after birth. While cerebral palsy is not a genetic disorder, it can be associated with genetic risk factors that make a child more vulnerable to brain injury. Children with cerebral palsy often experience delays in reaching motor milestones, such as sitting, crawling, or walking, and may require physical therapy to improve their mobility.

In addition to these specific genetic disorders, other genetic abnormalities, such as chromosomal deletions or duplication, can also contribute to developmental delays. Advances in genetic testing, such as chromosomal micro-array analysis and whole-exhume sequencing, have made it easier to identify genetic causes of developmental delays, providing families with more information about their child's condition and potential treatment options.

Biological factors, including brain injuries or infections that affect the developing brain, can also result in developmental delays. For example, traumatic brain injuries (TBI) caused by accidents or abuse can lead to cognitive, motor, and emotional impairments that affect a child's ability to develop normally. Similarly, infections such as meningitis or encephalitis can cause inflammation of the brain, leading to long-term developmental delays.

Premature is another biological factor that can increase the risk of developmental delays. Babies born before 37 weeks of gestation are at higher risk for neurological complications, which can affect their cognitive and motor development. Premature infants often experience delays in reaching physical milestones, such as walking or sitting up, and may require ongoing medical and developmental support.

Environmental Influences

While genetic and biological factors play a significant role in developmental delays, environmental influences can also have a profound impact on a child's development. The environment in which a child is raised—including the quality of care giving, access to educational opportunities, and exposure to toxic substances—can either support or hinder their growth.

Poverty is one of the most significant environmental risk factors associated with developmental delays. Children growing up in low-income households are more likely to experience delays in language, cognitive, and social-emotional development. Poverty often limits access to high-quality early education, healthcare, and nutrition, all of which are critical for healthy development. Additionally, parents living in poverty may experience higher levels of stress and have fewer resources to provide stimulating learning environments for their children. This can result in fewer opportunities for early language development, play, and social interaction, all of which are essential for reaching developmental milestones.

Toxic stress is another environmental factor that can negatively affect a child's development. Toxic stress refers to prolonged exposure to adverse experiences, such as neglect, abuse, or chronic household instability (e.g., parental substance abuse or domestic violence). These experiences can disrupt the developing brain and result in long-term developmental delays. Children exposed to toxic stress may experience delays in emotional regulation, social skills, and cognitive abilities, and are at higher risk for behavioral problems and mental health issues later in life.

Exposure to environmental toxins during early childhood can also lead to developmental delays. For example, lead exposure has been linked to delays in cognitive development, language impairments, and behavioral issues. Lead exposure often occurs in homes with lead-based paint or contaminated water, and children are particularly vulnerable to its effects because their brains are still developing. Other environmental toxins, such as mercury or pesticides, can also harm a child's brain development and result in delays across multiple domains.

In contrast, a stimulating and nurturing environment can support healthy development and help prevent delays. Children who grow up in environments rich with language, play, and social interaction are more likely to reach their developmental milestones on time. Positive parental involvement, such as talking, reading, and playing with a child, promotes cognitive and language development, while secure attachment to caregivers supports emotional regulation and social skills. Early childhood education programs, such as preschool and Head Start, also provide structured learning environments that help children develop important cognitive and social-emotional skills, reducing the risk of delays.

Prenatal and Birth Complications

The prenatal period, from conception to birth, is a critical time for a child's development. Factors that affect the fetus during this time, including maternal health, prenatal care, and birth complications, can have long-lasting effects on a child's development. Prenatal and birth complications are common causes of developmental delays, and in some cases, these delays may not become apparent until the child reaches toddler hood or preschool age.

Maternal health during pregnancy plays a significant role in a child's development. Maternal illnesses or infections, such as rubella, cytomegalovirus (CMV), or Zika virus, can interfere with fetal brain development and lead to developmental delays. For example, children exposed to the Zika virus in utero may be born with microcephaly, a condition in which the brain is underdeveloped, leading to cognitive and motor impairments. Maternal infections can also increase the risk of premature birth, which is associated with a higher likelihood of developmental delays.

Substance use during pregnancy is another major risk factor for developmental delays. Exposure to alcohol, tobacco, or illicit drugs in utero can lead to a range of developmental problems, including physical abnormalities, intellectual disabilities, and behavioral issues. Fetal Alcohol Spectrum

Disorders (FASD), caused by prenatal alcohol exposure, are a leading cause of intellectual disability and developmental delays. Children with FASD may experience delays in language, social skills, and cognitive development, as well as difficulties with attention and impulse control.

Birth complications can also result in developmental delays. For example, prolonged labor or complications during delivery, such as oxygen deprivation (hypoxia), can lead to brain injuries that affect a child's ability to reach developmental milestones. Cerebral palsy, a neurological disorder that affects movement and coordination, is often caused by birth complications that result in brain damage. Children with cerebral palsy may experience delays in motor skills, such as crawling, walking, and grasping objects, and may require physical therapy to improve their mobility.

Premature, as mentioned earlier, is a significant risk factor for developmental delays. Babies born prematurely are more likely to experience complications such as brain bleeds (intraventricular hemorrhage), respiratory distress, and feeding difficulties, all of which can affect their development. In particular, babies born before 28 weeks of gestation (extremely preterm) are at the highest risk for developmental delays, including intellectual disabilities, language impairments, and motor skill deficits.

Low birth weight is another risk factor associated with developmental delays. Babies who are born weighing less than 5.5 pounds are more likely to experience delays in physical growth, motor skills, and cognitive development. Low birth weight is often a result of premature birth, but it can also occur in full-term infants who experience growth restrictions in the womb. These infants may require additional medical care and developmental support during the first few years of life to help them catch up to their peers.

Nutrition and Early Childhood Health

Proper nutrition is essential for healthy brain and body development, particularly during the first few years of life. In early childhood, the brain is rapidly developing, and it requires adequate nutrition to support this process. Nutritional deficiencies, particularly during critical periods of growth, can lead to long-term developmental delays. This section will explore the role of nutrition and early childhood health in influencing developmental outcomes, and how both deficiencies and proper nourishment can shape a child's development.

Nutritional deficiencies are a common cause of developmental delays, particularly in low-income populations or areas where access to a balanced diet is limited. The most critical nutrients for brain development include iron, iodine, omega-3 fatty acids, and various vitamins, such as vitamins A, D, and B12. Deficiencies in any of these essential nutrients can have significant negative effects on a child's cognitive, motor, and social-emotional development.

1. Iron deficiency is one of the most common nutritional deficiencies in young children and is particularly problematic for brain development. Iron is crucial for oxygen transport in the blood and for brain function. Children with iron deficiency anemia often experience delays in cognitive development, including difficulties with attention, memory, and learning. Iron deficiency can also lead to fatigue, which may reduce a child's ability to engage in physical activities and social interactions. Studies have shown that children who are iron-deficient in early childhood are more likely to experience long-term cognitive and behavioral impairments, even after their iron levels are corrected.

2. Iodine deficiency is another major concern, particularly in areas where iodized salt is not widely available. Iodine is necessary for the production of thyroid hormones, which regulate brain development and growth. A lack of iodine during pregnancy and early childhood can lead to cretinism, a condition characterized by severe intellectual disability and stunted physical growth. Even mild iodine deficiency has been linked to lower IQ scores

and developmental delays in children. Ensuring that pregnant women and young children have access to iodine-rich foods or supplements is essential for preventing these outcomes.

3. Omega-3 fatty acids, particularly docosahexaenoic acid (DHA), are critical for brain development and function. Omega-3s play a role in building cell membranes in the brain and promoting communication between neurons. Studies have shown that children who consume diets rich in omega-3s have better cognitive outcomes, including improved memory, problem-solving skills, and attention. Conversely, a lack of omega-3 fatty acids in the diet can contribute to developmental delays, particularly in cognitive and behavioral domains.

4. Vitamin deficiencies can also contribute to developmental delays. For example, a lack of vitamin D can impair bone development and lead to conditions such as rickets, which can affect gross motor development. Vitamin A deficiency, which is more common in developing countries, can lead to vision problems and immune system dysfunction, both of which can indirectly affect a child's ability to explore their environment and engage in learning. B12 deficiency, often seen in children with limited access to animal-based foods, can cause neurological problems, including developmental delays and difficulties with motor skills.

Ensuring that children receive adequate nutrition during early childhood is essential for supporting healthy development. This requires not only access to a balanced diet but also education for parents and caregivers about the importance of nutrition during these critical years. In many cases, nutritional supplements may be necessary to address deficiencies, particularly in areas where certain nutrients are not readily available in the diet.

In addition to nutritional factors, early childhood health plays a critical role in a child's development. Chronic illnesses and infections during infancy and early childhood can interfere with developmental progress and lead to delays.

For example, children who experience frequent ear infections (otitis media) may have difficulty hearing, which can lead to speech and language delays. Similarly, children with chronic respiratory problems, such as asthma, may have difficulty engaging in physical activities, which can delay gross motor development.

Immunizations are another important aspect of early childhood health that can help prevent developmental delays. Vaccines protect children from serious infections, such as measles, mumps, and rubella, which can cause brain damage and developmental regression if left untreated. Ensuring that children receive their recommended vaccinations on schedule is critical for preventing these infections and their potentially devastating effects on development.

Breastfeeding has also been shown to have a positive impact on child development. Breast milk contains essential nutrients, antibodies, and other factors that support healthy brain development and immune function. Research has consistently shown that breastfed infants tend to have better cognitive outcomes, including higher IQ scores and better school performance, compared to formula-fed infants. The World Health Organization (WHO) recommends exclusive breastfeeding for the first six months of life, followed by continued breastfeeding along with the introduction of solid foods for up to two years or beyond. Promoting breastfeeding and providing support for breastfeeding mothers can help ensure that infants receive the best possible start in life.

In addition to proper nutrition and preventive healthcare, early intervention services are crucial for addressing developmental delays in young children. Early intervention programs, such as speech therapy, occupational therapy, and physical therapy, provide targeted support for children with developmental delays and help them build the skills they need to catch up to their peers. These services are most effective when they are initiated early, which is why regular developmental screenings and well-child visits are essential for identifying children who may need extra support.

Parents and caregivers play a key role in promoting healthy development by providing a safe, nurturing environment for their children. Parental involvement is critical for ensuring that children receive the proper nutrition, healthcare, and developmental support they need. Parents are encouraged to engage with their children through activities such as reading, talking, and playing, all of which promote cognitive, language, and social-emotional development. In addition, parents should be proactive in seeking help if they notice any signs of developmental delays in their child, as early intervention can make a significant difference in long-term outcomes.

Understanding the causes of developmental delays is essential for preventing and addressing these challenges in early childhood. Genetic and biological factors, environmental influences, prenatal and birth complications, and nutrition all play a role in shaping a child's development. By recognizing these factors and taking steps to mitigate their effects, parents, caregivers, and healthcare professionals can help ensure that children reach their full developmental potential. Early identification and intervention, combined with a nurturing and supportive environment, are key to helping children with developmental delays thrive.

Early Interventions and Why They Matter

E arly intervention refers to the services and supports that are provided to infants, toddlers, and young children who exhibit developmental delays or disabilities. The importance of early intervention cannot be overstated, as research consistently demonstrates that addressing developmental challenges as early as possible leads to improved outcomes in cognitive, physical, and social-emotional development. Early interventions are grounded in the principle that the earlier a child receives help, the more likely they are to overcome delays and avoid long-term challenges.

In this chapter, we explore the benefits of early interventions, discuss the critical timing and windows of opportunity for these services, and review evidence-based early intervention programs that have shown to be effective in supporting children with developmental delays. Understanding the value of early intervention can help parents, caregivers, and professionals take proactive steps to support the healthy development of children who may be at risk for delays.

Benefits of Early Interventions

The benefits of early intervention are profound and far-reaching, affecting multiple areas of a child's development. Early intervention services aim to provide children with the skills and tools they need to function more effectively in their daily lives and to catch up with their peers in areas where they may be lagging. These benefits extend not only to the child but also to their families and communities.

One of the most significant benefits of early intervention is its ability to improve cognitive development. Children who receive early intervention services show marked improvements in their ability to think, learn, and problem-solve. This is especially true for children who receive interventions targeting specific areas of cognitive delay, such as attention, memory, and executive function. For example, speech and language therapy can help children with communication delays develop the skills needed to express themselves and understand others, which in turn supports cognitive growth by enhancing their ability to interact with the world around them.

In addition to cognitive gains, early intervention is known to significantly enhance social and emotional development. Children with developmental delays often struggle with social skills, emotional regulation, and forming relationships with peers and adults. Early interventions that focus on these areas, such as play therapy or social skills training, can help children learn how to navigate social situations, regulate their emotions, and build positive relationships with others. This not only improves their immediate social interactions but also lays the foundation for future success in school and other social settings.

Motor skill development is another area where early intervention can make a dramatic difference. For children with gross or fine motor delays, physical and occupational therapies are essential in helping them build strength, coordination, and dexterity. These therapies focus on improving a child's ability to perform everyday tasks, such as walking, running, holding objects, and manipulating tools like pencils or scissors. As a result, children who receive early intervention in this area are more likely to develop the physical skills needed for independence and academic success.

Moreover, early intervention has been shown to reduce the need for more intensive services later in life. By addressing developmental challenges early on, children are less likely to require special education services, long-term therapy, or other supports as they grow older. This not only reduces the burden on families but also leads to significant cost savings for educational and healthcare systems.

Early intervention also offers substantial benefits for families. Parenting a child with developmental delays can be challenging, and many parents experience stress, frustration, and uncertainty as they navigate their child's needs. Early intervention services often include family-centered approaches, providing parents with the guidance, resources, and support they need to help their child succeed. This includes training parents on how to implement intervention strategies at home, as well as offering counseling or support groups for families coping with the emotional and practical challenges of raising a child with developmental delays. As a result, early intervention helps strengthen family relationships and improves the overall well-being of both the child and their caregivers.

Timing and Windows of Opportunity

The timing of early intervention is crucial, as there are specific windows of opportunity during which a child's brain is most receptive to change and growth. These windows are periods of heightened neuroplasticity, meaning the brain is more adaptable and can form new connections more easily in response to experiences and interventions. This is why the earliest years of life—particularly the first three years—are so critical for development.

During early childhood, a child's brain is undergoing rapid growth and development. Neurons are forming new connections, and existing pathways are being strengthened or pruned based on the child's experiences. This process is most active during infancy and toddler hood, making this period a prime time for interventions that target developmental delays. For example, research has shown that children who receive early language interventions are more likely to develop the communication skills needed for academic success, as the brain's language centers are highly plastic during this time.

The concept of neuroplasticity underscores the importance of providing interventions during these early years. When a child experiences delays in any area of development—whether in language, motor skills, or social-emotional functioning—early intervention takes advantage of the brain's natural ability to adapt. By providing targeted support during this critical window, early intervention can help "re-wire" the brain in ways that promote healthier development and allow the child to catch up to their peers.

Missing these early windows of opportunity can result in more entrenched developmental challenges that are harder to overcome later in life. For example, a child who experiences significant speech and language delays during the early years may struggle with reading and writing in school, which can lead to long-term academic difficulties. Similarly, delays in social-emotional development can result in behavioral problems and difficulties forming relationships, which may persist into adolescence and adulthood if not addressed early on.

Timing is also crucial for children with more complex developmental disorders, such as autism spectrum disorder (ASD) or intellectual disabilities. Research shows that children with ASD who receive early intervention—often before the age of three—demonstrate significant improvements in communication, social skills, and behavior compared to children who receive interventions later. Early behavioral therapies, such as applied behavior analysis (ABA), are particularly effective when implemented during the early stages of brain development, as they help shape the child's social and communication skills before more rigid patterns of behavior become established.

In addition to targeting the brain's natural plasticity, early intervention capitalizes on the sensitive periods in which specific developmental domains are most malleable. For example, the sensitive period for language development occurs during the first few years of life. Children who are exposed to rich language environments during this time are more likely to develop strong language skills, while children who lack this exposure may experience lasting language delays. Early intervention programs that provide speech therapy or language-enriching activities during this window can make a significant difference in a child's long-term communication abilities.

While early intervention is most effective when implemented during these sensitive periods, it is important to note that it is never too late to begin addressing developmental delays. Even after the first three years of life, children can benefit from interventions that support their growth and development. However, the earlier these services are initiated, the greater the potential for positive outcomes.

Evidence-Based Early Intervention Programs

There are a wide variety of early intervention programs designed to address different types of developmental delays. These programs are grounded in research and evidence-based practices, meaning they have been rigorously tested and proven to be effective in improving developmental outcomes for children. Evidence-based programs often target specific areas of delay, such as language, motor skills, or social-emotional development, and are tailored to meet the individual needs of each child.

One of the most well-known early intervention programs is Early Intervention (EI), a federally funded program in the United States that provides services to children from birth to three years of age who are experiencing developmental delays or disabilities. Early Intervention services are available in every state and are tailored to the unique needs of each child and family. The program typically includes a wide range of services, such as speech therapy, physical therapy, occupational therapy, and developmental support, all aimed at helping children reach their developmental milestones.

The Early Start Denver Model (ESDM) is another evidence-based early intervention program that is specifically designed for young children with autism spectrum disorder (ASD). ESDM is a comprehensive, play-based program that incorporates both behavioral and developmental approaches to improve communication, social interaction, and cognitive skills. It is typically implemented with children between 12 and 48 months of age and has been shown to produce significant gains in language, social engagement, and cognitive functioning. ESDM is unique in that it can be delivered in both home and clinic settings, allowing for greater flexibility in meeting the needs of each child and family.

Applied Behavior Analysis (ABA) is another widely recognized early intervention program, particularly for children with autism. ABA focuses on teaching new skills and reducing challenging behaviors through positive reinforcement and structured learning experiences. The principles of ABA are rooted in behavioral psychology, and the program is highly individualized, with interventions tailored to each child's specific strengths and needs. ABA is often used to target communication skills, social interaction, and daily living skills, and it has been shown to be highly effective in helping children with autism make meaningful progress in these areas.

For children with motor skill delays, physical therapy and occupational therapy are key components of early intervention. Physical therapy focuses on improving gross motor skills, such as walking, running, and climbing, while occupational therapy targets fine motor skills, such as grasping objects, manipulating tools, and performing self-care tasks. These therapies are often provided in combination with other services, such as speech therapy or developmental support, to address the child's overall developmental needs.

Speech and language therapy is another critical component of early intervention for children with communication delays. Speech therapists work with children to improve their ability to understand and use language, develop social communication skills, and address any speech sound disorders or articulation issues. Early speech and language interventions are particularly important for children with developmental language disorder (DLD) or children with delays in expressive and receptive language. These therapies often incorporate play-based activities to engage the child and make learning more interactive and fun.

In addition to these therapies, early literacy programs are an important component of early intervention for children who show delays in language and cognitive development. These programs focus on building foundational skills for reading and writing, such as phonological awareness, vocabulary, and narrative skills. Early literacy programs often include activities like shared reading, storytelling, and language games that encourage children to engage with books and language in meaningful ways. These interventions not only support cognitive development but also foster a love of reading, which can have long-term benefits for academic success.

For children with social and emotional delays, evidence-based programs like The Incredible Years or Parent-Child Interaction Therapy (PCIT) are designed to improve social skills, emotional regulation, and behavior management. These programs focus on strengthening the parent-child relationship and teaching children how to interact with others in positive ways. The Incredible Years, for example, is a comprehensive program that includes group-based sessions for parents and children, teaching strategies for managing challenging behaviors, enhancing emotional regulation, and promoting positive social interactions. Parent-Child Interaction Therapy (PCIT) combines direct coaching of parents with live feedback on how they interact with their children, helping to improve both the child's behavior and the parent-child relationship.

Early Head Start, a federally funded program in the United States, provides comprehensive early childhood education, health, and social services to low-income families with children under the age of three. The program is designed to promote healthy development and school readiness by offering high-quality early education, health screenings, nutrition support, and family services. Research on Early Head Start has shown that children who participate in the program are more likely to meet developmental milestones and are better prepared for school than their peers who do not receive these services.

Play-based therapies, such as floor time or play therapy, are also widely used in early intervention to support children's social, emotional, and cognitive development. Play-based therapies allow children to express their emotions, explore their environment, and develop problem-solving skills through guided play. These therapies are particularly beneficial for children with autism, trauma, or emotional regulation challenges, as they provide a safe and structured environment for the child to work through their developmental challenges.

Family-centered interventions are a core principle of early intervention programs. These interventions emphasize the importance of involving parents and caregivers in the therapeutic process, recognizing that parents are the most important influence on their child's development. Family-centered programs often include parent training, support groups, and home-based services that help parents learn how to support their child's development in the home environment. By empowering parents with the knowledge and tools they need, family-centered interventions create a supportive and nurturing environment that promotes the child's progress and overall well-being.

In addition to structured programs, early intervention often includes multi-disciplinary teams of professionals who work together to address the child's developmental needs. These teams may include speech therapists, physical therapists, occupational therapists, psychologists, and special educators, all of whom collaborate to create an individualized plan for the child. This multi-disciplinary approach ensures that the child receives comprehensive care that addresses all areas of development, from motor skills and communication to cognitive and social-emotional growth.

Research shows that the most effective early intervention programs are those that are evidence-based, meaning they are supported by scientific research and have been proven to lead to positive outcomes for children with developmental delays. These programs are often evaluated through rigorous studies that measure their impact on children's development over time. The success of early intervention programs is also linked to their individualization—programs that are tailored to the specific needs of each child and family tend to be more effective than one-size-fits-all approaches.

Ultimately, the success of early intervention relies on early identification and referral. Pediatricians, caregivers, and educators play a key role in identifying children who may be at risk for developmental delays and referring them for evaluation and intervention services. Regular developmental screenings, as discussed in previous chapters, are essential for ensuring that children who need early intervention are identified as soon as possible. By catching delays early and providing timely, evidence-based interventions, we can help children overcome developmental challenges and set them on a path toward long-term success.

In , early intervention is a critical tool for addressing developmental delays and promoting healthy child development. The benefits of early intervention are wide-ranging, from improved cognitive and motor skills to enhanced social and emotional development. Early intervention takes advantage of the brain's plasticity during the critical early years of life, making it possible for children to overcome delays and reach their full potential. By implementing evidence-based early intervention programs, providing family-centered care, and ensuring timely access to services, we can make a significant difference in the lives of children with developmental delays, helping them thrive both in the short term and throughout their lives.

Speech and Language Interventions

S peech and language development is a cornerstone of a child's ability to communicate effectively and interact with the world around them. For many children with developmental delays, speech and language challenges can be some of the most difficult to overcome. Whether a child has difficulty forming words, understanding language, or using speech to communicate, speech therapy and other interventions can play a critical role in helping them reach their full communicative potential. This chapter will explore what to expect from speech therapy, strategies for supporting non-verbal children, and the tools and resources available for enhancing speech development.

Speech Therapy: What to Expect

Speech therapy is one of the most common interventions for children experiencing speech and language delays. The primary goal of speech therapy is to help children improve their ability to communicate, whether through verbal language, gestures, or other forms of communication. Speech therapy is highly individualized, with each therapy plan tailored to meet the specific needs of the child. It is typically conducted by licensed speech-language pathologists (SLPs) who are trained to assess and treat speech and language disorders in children.

The first step in speech therapy is a comprehensive assessment, during which the SLP evaluates the child's current abilities and identifies areas of difficulty.

This assessment may include a combination of observations, standardized tests, and input from parents or caregivers about the child's speech and language development. The results of the assessment are used to create a personalized treatment plan that outlines specific goals for the child. These goals may vary depending on the child's age and the nature of their speech and language challenges, but they typically focus on improving articulation, language comprehension, expressive language, or social communication.

In speech therapy sessions, children engage in a variety of activities designed to improve their communication skills. These activities are often play-based, especially for younger children, as play provides a natural context for language learning. For example, an SLP might use toys, picture books, or games to encourage a child to practice forming sounds, words, or sentences. For older children, therapy may involve more structured tasks, such as practicing specific speech sounds or working on language comprehension exercises. The therapist may also introduce visual or auditory aids, such as flashcards, speech-generating devices, or apps, to support the child's learning.

Articulation therapy is one of the most common forms of speech therapy, particularly for children with speech sound disorders. This type of therapy focuses on helping children produce specific speech sounds correctly. During articulation therapy, the SLP will model how to produce the sound and provide feedback to the child as they practice. For example, if a child has difficulty pronouncing the "r" sound, the therapist might guide them through exercises that help them position their tongue correctly and gradually improve their articulation of the sound in words and sentences.

Language therapy focuses on helping children improve their understanding and use of language. For children with receptive language delays, therapy might involve activities that help them follow directions, understand new vocabulary, or process questions and commands. For children with expressive language delays, therapy may focus on helping them form sentences, use correct grammar, or expand their vocabulary. Language therapy also often includes social communication skills, such as taking turns in conversation, maintaining eye contact, and using language appropriately in different social contexts.

Children with apraxia of speech, a motor speech disorder that affects the ability to plan and produce speech movements, may require a different type of therapy known as motor planning therapy. This approach focuses on helping children practice the precise movements needed to produce speech sounds. The SLP may use repetitive exercises, such as saying the same word or sound multiple times, to help the child develop more accurate speech production.

Parents and caregivers are an integral part of the speech therapy process. SLPs often work closely with families to provide guidance on how to support their child's communication development at home. This may include providing specific exercises or activities for parents to practice with their child between therapy sessions, as well as offering strategies for improving communication in everyday situations. For example, parents might be encouraged to narrate their daily activities to help expose their child to new vocabulary, or to use gestures or pictures to reinforce spoken language.

Speech therapy can take place in a variety of settings, including clinics, schools, or even the child's home. The frequency and duration of therapy sessions vary depending on the child's needs, but many children benefit from regular, ongoing therapy over the course of several months or years. Progress in speech therapy can be gradual, and it is important for parents and caregivers to remain patient and supportive as their child works toward their communication goals.

Communication Strategies for Non-Verbal Children

For some children, verbal speech may not be their primary mode of communi-cation, either temporarily or permanently. These children are often described as non-verbal or minimally verbal and may have difficulty producing speech sounds or using spoken language to communicate. However, being non-verbal does not mean that a child is unable to communicate. In fact, there are many alternative communication strategies that can help non-verbal children express their needs, thoughts, and emotions effectively.

One of the most widely used strategies for non-verbal communication is augmentative and alternative communication (AAC). AAC encompasses a range of communication methods that support or replace verbal speech, including gestures, sign language, picture-based communication systems, and speech-generating devices. AAC can be used as a temporary support while a child develops verbal speech or as a long-term solution for children who are unable to use spoken language.

Sign language is one form of AAC that can be particularly beneficial for non-verbal children. Teaching a child basic signs, such as those for "eat," "drink," or "help," can provide them with a way to communicate their needs before they are able to use spoken language. Many non-verbal children find it easier to use their hands to sign than to produce speech sounds, and learning sign language can reduce frustration by giving them an immediate way to express themselves. In some cases, children who use sign language eventually develop spoken language skills, as the use of signs helps build their understanding of communication.

Another common AAC strategy is the use of picture exchange communication systems (PECS). PECS is a communication system in which a child uses picture cards to represent objects, actions, or concepts. The child can use these picture cards to make requests or share information with others. For example, if a child wants a drink, they might hand a picture of a cup to their caregiver. Over time, the child can learn to use more complex combinations of pictures to communicate full sentences or express more abstract ideas.

Speech-generating devices (SGDs) are another option for non-verbal children. These devices, sometimes referred to as "communication devices," allow a child to select words, phrases, or sentences on a touchscreen or keyboard, which the device then "speaks" aloud. SGDs can be highly customization, allowing the user to select vocabulary that is most relevant to their needs and interests. These devices are particularly helpful for children with physical or neurological conditions that make it difficult to produce speech sounds, as they provide a way for the child to participate in conversations and express themselves verbally through technology.

In addition to AAC, there are several other strategies that parents and care-givers can use to support non-verbal children's communication development. Visual supports, such as visual schedules or communication boards, can help non-verbal children understand routines, make choices, and communicate their needs. For example, a visual schedule might include pictures of daily activities, such as eating breakfast, going to school, or playing, which the child can point to in order to indicate their preferences or needs.

It is important to remember that every child is different, and what works for one non-verbal child may not work for another. Some children may prefer using gestures or sign language, while others may benefit more from picture-based communication systems or speech-generating devices. The key is to provide the child with a communication system that is accessible, meaningful, and tailored to their individual abilities and needs.

Parents and caregivers can also use modeling to support non-verbal communi-cation. This involves demonstrating the use of AAC or other communication strategies while interacting with the child. For example, if a parent is using PECS with their child, they might model how to use the picture cards to make requests by selecting a card themselves and showing the child how it works. Modeling helps the child understand that their communication system is a valid and effective way to interact with others, and it encourages them to use the system consistently.

Incorporating play-based communication is another effective strategy for non-verbal children. Play provides a natural context for communication and helps children practice using their AAC systems in a low-pressure environment. For example, a caregiver might set up a pretend tea party and encourage the child to use their communication device to request items or direct the play. Engaging in play helps reinforce communication skills while also providing opportunities for social interaction and language learning.

Tools and Resources for Speech Development

In addition to speech therapy and AAC strategies, there are numerous tools and resources available to support speech and language development in children with delays. These tools can be used at home, in therapy sessions, or in educational settings to enhance a child's communication skills and promote language growth.

Apps and digital tools have become increasingly popular for supporting speech development in children. Many speech therapy apps are designed to target specific speech and language skills, such as articulation, phonological awareness, or sentence construction. For example, apps like Articulation Station and Speech Blubs provide interactive exercises that help children practice producing specific speech sounds in a fun and engaging way. Other apps, like Proloquo2Go, serve as communication devices for non-verbal children, allowing them to select words or phrases from a digital interface that "speaks" for them.

Parents and caregivers can also use interactive books to support speech development. Books that encourage children to participate by naming objects, repeating words, or making sounds can help reinforce language learning. Many speech therapists recommend books with simple, repetitive text or predictable patterns that encourage children to anticipate and produce language. For example, books like Brown Bear, Brown Bear, What Do You See? or Goodnight Moon provide opportunities for children to practice naming animals, colors, or objects, while the repetitive structure helps reinforce language patterns. Interactive books that allow children to lift flaps, press buttons, or manipulate movable parts can also engage them in ways that promote both language and motor skill development.

Flashcards and visual aids are another valuable resource for supporting speech development. Flashcards with pictures of everyday objects, animals, or actions can help children build their vocabulary by associating words with images. These cards can be used in a variety of ways, such as having the child point to or name the object, or matching the picture with a spoken word. Flashcards are particularly helpful for children with receptive language delays, as they provide a visual representation of the words they are learning. For children with expressive language delays, flashcards can be used to practice forming sentences, describing the picture, or asking and answering questions.

Speech therapy toys and games can also be effective tools for encouraging speech and language development. Toys that require turn-taking, problem-solving, or imaginative play help create opportunities for communication. For example, board games that require players to describe what they see, follow directions, or ask for help can promote language use in a fun and natural way. Building blocks, puzzles, and playsets like dollhouses or farms can also be used to practice vocabulary, sentence construction, and conversation skills as children describe their actions, narrate a story, or engage in pretend play.

Social stories are another resource that can be particularly helpful for children with social communication challenges. Social stories are short, simple narratives that explain social situations or concepts in a way that is accessible to children. For example, a social story might explain how to take turns in conversation, how to ask for help, or what to expect during a doctor's visit. These stories often include pictures or symbols to help reinforce the language and concepts being taught. Social stories can be used to help children understand and practice social communication skills in a low-pressure setting before applying them in real-life situations.

Songs and rhymes can also be powerful tools for speech development. Music provides a rhythmic and engaging way for children to learn language, as the repetition and melody make it easier for them to remember and produce words. Songs with actions or gestures, such as "The Wheels on the Bus" or "Itsy Bitsy Spider," combine language learning with motor skill development, as children sing along and imitate the movements. Rhymes, finger plays, and nursery rhymes are also effective for developing phonological awareness, as they draw attention to the sounds and patterns in words, helping children with speech sound production and early literacy skills.

Parent training programs are another valuable resource for supporting speech and language development. These programs provide parents and caregivers with the tools and strategies they need to promote language growth at home. Programs like Hanen's It Takes Two to Talk are designed to teach parents how to interact with their child in ways that encourage communication, whether through play, daily routines, or reading together. Parent training programs emphasize the importance of creating language-rich environments, responding to the child's communication attempts, and modeling appropriate language use. By empowering parents with knowledge and strategies, these programs help create a supportive home environment that fosters speech and language development.

Collaborative support from educators is also essential for children with speech and language delays, especially as they enter preschool or elementary school. Many children with communication challenges receive speech therapy as part of their individualized education program (IEP) or through school-based speech-language services. Teachers and speech therapists work together to create a language-rich classroom environment and provide accommodations or modifications to support the child's learning. For example, a child with a speech sound disorder may be given extra time to respond during classroom discussions, or a child with language comprehension difficulties may receive visual supports to help them understand instructions. In addition to formal therapy sessions, teachers can incorporate language-building activities into the classroom, such as group discussions, storytelling, and interactive games.

Finally, community resources such as local speech therapy clinics, early intervention programs, and support groups for parents of children with developmental delays provide additional support for families seeking speech and language interventions. Early intervention programs, such as those offered through public health departments or school systems, provide comprehensive services for children under the age of three who are experiencing developmental delays. These programs often include speech therapy as well as other services like physical or occupational therapy, depending on the child's needs. Many communities also offer support groups or workshops where parents can connect with others facing similar challenges, share resources, and learn strategies for supporting their child's development.

In , speech and language interventions are crucial for helping children overcome communication challenges and achieve their full potential. Through a combination of speech therapy, alternative communication strategies, and a wide array of tools and resources, children with speech and language delays can make significant progress in their ability to understand and use language. Whether through individualized therapy sessions, AAC devices, or interactive games and books, there are numerous ways to support a child's speech development and enhance their communication skills. With the right interventions and support, children with speech and language delays can build the foundation they need for success in school, social relationships, and beyond.

Motor Skills Interventions

Motor skills are essential for a child's ability to explore the world, interact with their environment, and perform daily tasks. They are generally divided into two categories: fine motor skills, which involve the coordination of small muscles in movements like grasping or manipulating objects, and gross motor skills, which involve larger muscle groups responsible for activities such as walking, running, and jumping. When children experience developmental delays or impairments in motor skills, it can significantly impact their ability to engage in everyday activities, including self-care, play, and learning. Early intervention through occupational and physical therapy, as well as targeted exercises and activities, can help children improve both fine and gross motor skills, enabling them to gain greater independence and confidence in their abilities.

Motor skill delays are common in children with developmental disorders, including cerebral palsy, autism spectrum disorder (ASD), Down syndrome, and other genetic or neurological conditions. These delays may also occur in children who have experienced birth complications, traumatic injuries, or health conditions that affect the brain or muscles. In some cases, children may simply exhibit motor delays without a clear underlying cause. Regardless of the reason, motor skill interventions play a crucial role in helping children overcome these challenges and develop the physical abilities necessary for everyday functioning.

Occupational Therapy for Fine Motor Skills

Occupational therapy (OT) focuses on helping children develop the fine motor skills they need to perform activities of daily living (ADLs), such as dressing, feeding, writing, and using tools or utensils. Fine motor skills are critical for tasks that require precision and control, such as holding a pencil, tying shoelaces, or buttoning a shirt. Occupational therapists work with children to improve hand-eye coordination, dexterity, strength, and other key aspects of fine motor control.

The first step in occupational therapy is a thorough assessment of the child's current abilities and challenges. Occupational therapists use standardized assessments, observations, and input from parents and teachers to identify areas where the child is struggling. For example, a child may have difficulty holding a pencil properly, cutting with scissors, or manipulating small objects like building blocks. Based on this assessment, the therapist develops a customized intervention plan that targets the child's specific needs.

One of the primary goals of occupational therapy is to improve hand strength and dexterity. Weakness in the hands or fingers can make it difficult for children to perform tasks that require precision, such as writing or using utensils. To address this, occupational therapists often incorporate a variety of exercises and activities designed to strengthen the muscles in the hands and fingers. These may include tasks like squeezing putty, using tweezers to pick up small objects, or threading beads onto a string. Over time, these activities help improve grip strength, finger control, and overall dexterity.

Another important focus of occupational therapy is improving hand-eye coordination. Many fine motor tasks, such as catching a ball or writing on a line, require the child to coordinate their hand movements with visual input. Occupational therapists use activities like tracing shapes, playing with pegboards, or stacking blocks to help children practice these skills. By gradually increasing the difficulty of the tasks, therapists help children develop greater control over their movements and improve their ability to complete tasks that require precise coordination.

For children with sensory processing issues, occupational therapy may also include strategies for addressing tactile defensiveness or sensory-seeking behaviors. Some children with motor skill delays may be overly sensitive to touch, making it uncomfortable for them to handle certain textures or materials. Others may seek out sensory input by constantly touching or manipulating objects. Occupational therapists use sensory integration therapy to help children become more comfortable with different sensations and develop appropriate responses to sensory input. This might involve exposing the child to various textures (such as sand, rice, or soft fabrics) in a controlled and supportive environment, gradually helping them become more tolerant of these sensations.

For children with fine motor delays, occupational therapy often emphasizes self-care skills, such as dressing, grooming, and feeding. These skills are essential for promoting independence and enabling children to take care of themselves as they grow older. Occupational therapists use adaptive techniques and tools to help children practice these tasks in a way that matches their current abilities. For example, a child who has difficulty using a spoon may practice with a larger, easier-to-hold spoon, or a child who struggles with zippers may work on fastening larger zippers before moving on to more challenging ones. The therapist's goal is to break down complex tasks into manageable steps, helping the child build confidence and competence over time.

Occupational therapy sessions are typically play-based, particularly for younger children. By incorporating toys, games, and other engaging activities, therapists make therapy sessions fun and motivating for the child. For example, a therapist might use a fishing game to help a child practice using a pincer grip, or they might have the child complete a puzzle that requires manipulating small pieces. Play-based therapy not only helps improve fine motor skills but also supports the child's cognitive and social development by encouraging problem-solving, creativity, and interaction with others.

Parents and caregivers are a critical part of the occupational therapy process. Therapists often provide families with home-based activities and exercises that they can practice with their child between therapy sessions. These activities help reinforce the skills the child is learning in therapy and ensure that progress continues outside of the clinical setting. For example, parents might be encouraged to play with modeling clay, encourage their child to color or draw, or practice dressing skills like buttoning and zipping during their daily routine.

Physical Therapy for Gross Motor Skills

While occupational therapy focuses on fine motor skills, physical therapy (PT) is the primary intervention for children who have delays in gross motor skills, which involve the use of larger muscle groups for activities like crawling, walking, running, and jumping. Physical therapists work with children to improve their balance, coordination, strength, and mobility, helping them develop the skills they need for physical activities and independent movement.

As with occupational therapy, physical therapy begins with a comprehensive assessment of the child's motor abilities. The therapist evaluates the child's posture, muscle tone, range of motion, and ability to perform gross motor tasks like standing, walking, or climbing stairs. Based on this assessment, the therapist creates an individualized treatment plan that addresses the child's specific challenges.

One of the key goals of physical therapy is to improve balance and coordination, which are essential for many gross motor activities. Children with motor delays may have difficulty maintaining their balance while walking or standing, making it harder for them to participate in activities like playing on the playground, riding a bike, or even walking on uneven surfaces. Physical therapists use exercises like standing on one foot, walking on a balance beam, or hopping on one leg to help children practice these skills. These activities not only improve balance but also strengthen the muscles needed for stable and coordinated movement.

Strengthening exercises are another important component of physical therapy. Children with gross motor delays may have weak muscles, particularly in their core, legs, or arms, which can make it difficult for them to perform activities like running, jumping, or climbing. Physical therapists design exercises that target specific muscle groups, gradually increasing the intensity of the exercises as the child builds strength. For example, a therapist might have a child practice squats, push-ups, or lunges to improve leg and core strength, or they might use resistance bands or therapy balls to add an extra challenge to the exercises.

In addition to strength and balance, coordination is a key focus of physical therapy. Many gross motor activities, such as throwing a ball, riding a bike, or catching, require the child to coordinate multiple muscle groups and body parts. Physical therapists use activities like ball games, obstacle courses, or jumping exercises to help children improve their coordination. These exercises are designed to be fun and engaging, encouraging the child to practice their skills while also enjoying physical activity.

For children with cerebral palsy or other neurological conditions that affect motor function, physical therapy may also focus on improving mobility and range of motion. Children with cerebral palsy often experience tight muscles, spasticity, or joint stiffness, which can limit their ability to move freely. Physical therapists use stretching exercises and range-of-motion activities to help increase flexibility and reduce muscle tightness. They may also use equipment like braces, walkers, or wheelchairs to help children move more independently. The goal of physical therapy for these children is to maximize their mobility and improve their ability to participate in physical activities to the best of their abilities.

Gait training is another important aspect of physical therapy for children who have difficulty walking or have an abnormal gait pattern. Children with motor delays may walk with a limp, have difficulty maintaining a steady pace, or need assistance to walk. Physical therapists use gait training exercises to help children improve their walking pattern, balance, and endurance. This might involve practicing walking on different surfaces, using parallel bars for support, or working on stepping over obstacles. Over time, gait training can help children develop a more stable occupational and physical therapy sessions, children with motor skill delays can benefit greatly from exercises and activities that are designed to strengthen their motor skills at home or in other natural environments. These activities are typically play-based and fun, making them appealing to children while also promoting the development of both fine and gross motor skills. Regular practice of these exercises can help children build strength, improve coordination, and enhance their ability to perform everyday tasks more independently.

Fine Motor Skill Activities

Fine motor skills require precise control of small muscles, especially in the hands and fingers, and are necessary for tasks such as writing, buttoning, and using utensils. Strengthening fine motor skills involves activities that require children to manipulate objects, practice hand-eye coordination, and develop dexterity.

1. Play dough and Modeling Clay: One of the simplest and most effective ways to strengthen fine motor skills is through the use of play dough or modeling clay. Squeezing, rolling, and shaping the clay helps improve hand strength and finger dexterity. Children can create different shapes, cut the clay with child-safe scissors, or use cookie cutters to make patterns, all of which help improve their motor control and coordination.

2. Threading Beads or Lacing Cards: Threading small beads onto a string or using lacing cards is a great way to improve a child's ability to manipulate small objects, an important component of fine motor development. These activities help improve the child's grip strength and precision while also

enhancing their hand-eye coordination.

3. Puzzles and Pegboards: Completing puzzles and using pegboards are excellent activities for building fine motor skills. Puzzles with large pieces are ideal for younger children, while more complex puzzles or pegboards with small parts are appropriate for older children. These activities promote problem-solving skills and require the use of fine motor movements, such as picking up and placing puzzle pieces or pegs.

4. Cutting with Scissors: Practicing with child-safe scissors is another way to build fine motor strength and coordination. Children can start by cutting along straight lines on paper, and as they become more skilled, they can progress to cutting out shapes or following more complex patterns. This activity strengthens the muscles needed for writing and other precise hand movements.

5. Drawing, Coloring, and Writing: Encouraging children to engage in drawing or coloring helps them practice using a pincer grip (the ability to hold a pencil or crayon between the thumb and forefinger). Writing practice, whether through tracing letters or writing independently, also helps develop hand strength and fine motor control. Providing a variety of drawing tools, such as markers, crayons, and chalk, allows the child to explore different textures and grips.

6. Building with Blocks or Legos: Building with blocks or small interlocking pieces like Legos promotes fine motor development by requiring children to grasp, stack, and manipulate objects with precision. These activities not only strengthen fine motor skills but also encourage creativity, spatial awareness, and problem-solving.

Gross Motor Skill Activities

Gross motor skills involve the coordination of large muscle groups, particularly those in the legs, arms, and torso. These skills are essential for movement, balance, and overall physical coordination. Strengthening gross motor skills typically involves activities that promote full-body movement, balance, and endurance.

1. Obstacle Courses: Setting up a simple obstacle course with household items (such as cushions, chairs, and cones) provides children with the opportunity to practice a range of gross motor skills, including crawling, jumping, balancing, and climbing. Navigating the course requires the child to use strength, coordination, and spatial awareness, and it can be adapted to suit the child's skill level.

2. Ball Games: Playing with balls helps children develop hand-eye coordination, balance, and gross motor skills. Simple games like catching and throwing a ball, kicking a soccer ball, or dribbling a basketball are fun ways to build motor strength. For younger children or those with significant delays, starting with larger, lightweight balls can make these activities easier and more manageable.

3. Jumping Activities: Jumping is a key gross motor skill that strengthens the muscles in the legs and improves coordination. Activities like jumping over objects, playing hopscotch, or using a trampoline can help children practice jumping. Additionally, these activities enhance balance and coordination while providing a fun and engaging way to build muscle strength.

4. Balance Beam or Walking on Lines: Practicing balance by walking on a narrow surface (such as a balance beam or a line drawn on the ground) is an excellent way to improve coordination and stability. For younger children, starting with a wide line or low beam is ideal, and as their balance improves, the difficulty can be increased by narrowing the line or raising the beam.

5. Bicycle or Tricycle Riding: Riding a tricycle or bicycle is a great way for children to strengthen their leg muscles and improve coordination. Balancing on a bike, steering, and pedaling simultaneously requires the use of multiple

muscle groups, making it a comprehensive gross motor activity. Training wheels or balance bikes are useful for children who are just beginning to learn how to ride.

6. Climbing and Playground Equipment: Engaging in activities on playground equipment, such as climbing ladders, swinging on monkey bars, or sliding down slides, helps children develop upper and lower body strength as well as coordination. These activities challenge children to use their muscles in different ways while also improving their balance and flexibility.

7. Dancing or Yoga: Movement-based activities like dancing or practicing yoga can be both fun and beneficial for motor skill development. Dancing encourages rhythm, coordination, and balance, while yoga helps improve flexibility, strength, and body awareness. Simple yoga poses or dance routines can be adapted for children with varying abilities, making these activities accessible to all.

Incorporating Motor Skills Activities into Daily Routines

One of the most effective ways to strengthen motor skills is by incorporating targeted activities into a child's daily routine. This can be done through play, household chores, or structured exercise routines. For example, encouraging a child to help with tasks like sweeping, carrying groceries, or watering plants promotes gross motor strength, while activities like setting the table or sorting laundry can help build fine motor coordination.

Parents and caregivers can also integrate motor skill exercises into everyday play by offering toys and activities that promote physical engagement. For example, placing toys just out of reach can encourage a child to crawl or walk toward them, while playing with stacking blocks or sorting objects can provide fine motor practice.

The key to success in motor skill development is consistency and repetition. By regularly engaging in activities that target both fine and gross motor skills, children can build strength, coordination, and confidence in their physical abilities. Whether through occupational and physical therapy, home-based exercises, or playful activities, motor skill interventions help children overcome developmental challenges and achieve greater independence in their daily lives.

With the support of skilled therapists and the involvement of parents and caregivers, children with motor skill delays can make significant progress in their ability to perform everyday tasks, participate in physical activities, and engage with their environment. These interventions not only improve motor abilities but also enhance the child's overall quality of life by promoting physical health, self-confidence, and a sense of accomplishment.

Cognitive and Learning Interventions

C ognitive development and learning are fundamental components of a child's growth, affecting their ability to reason, problem-solve, remember, and make sense of the world around them. When children experience delays in cognitive or learning development, they may struggle with processing information, paying attention, or acquiring new skills in academic and everyday contexts. Fortunately, a variety of interventions, including cognitive behavioral strategies, early learning methods, and individualized educational plans, are available to support children in overcoming these challenges.

Cognitive and learning interventions are particularly important for children diagnosed with learning disabilities, attention deficit hyperactivity disorder (ADHD), autism spectrum disorder (ASD), intellectual disabilities, or other conditions that impact cognition and learning. These interventions can be provided at home, in school, or through specialized therapy programs, and they aim to help children develop the skills they need to succeed academically and socially.

Cognitive Behavioral Interventions

Cognitive-behavioral interventions (CBIs) focus on improving the way children think, perceive, and respond to their environment. They are based on the principle that thoughts, emotions, and behaviors are interconnected and that modifying unhelpful patterns of thinking can lead to more positive emotional and behavioral outcomes. For children with cognitive delays or learning difficulties, cognitive behavioral interventions can help them develop more effective strategies for managing their emotions, behaviors, and thought processes in academic and social settings.

One of the most widely used cognitive-behavioral interventions for children is Cognitive Behavioral Therapy (CBT). Although traditionally used for treating anxiety, depression, and other mental health disorders, CBT has been adapted to support children with cognitive and learning challenges. CBT helps children recognize negative thought patterns—such as "I'm not smart enough to do this" or "I'll never learn"—and replace them with more positive, constructive ways of thinking. This shift in perspective not only improves a child's emotional well-being but also enhances their ability to tackle difficult tasks, engage in learning, and persevere through challenges.

CBT typically involves structured sessions in which the child works with a therapist to identify and modify unhelpful thoughts and behaviors. For example, a child who struggles with focus in school may learn to identify distractions and develop strategies for redirecting their attention back to their work. Alternatively, a child with a learning disability may work on breaking down tasks into smaller, manageable steps, which helps reduce feelings of overwhelm. The therapist may also teach relaxation techniques or coping strategies to manage frustration or anxiety, which are common among children who experience academic difficulties.

In addition to individual therapy, cognitive-behavioral interventions can be implemented through group-based programs in schools or therapeutic settings. These programs often focus on building specific cognitive skills, such as attention, working memory, or problem-solving, through structured activities and exercises. For example, children may engage in games that require them to practice paying attention to details, following multi-step instructions, or using logic to solve puzzles. Group-based interventions also offer opportunities for social learning, as children observe and learn from their peers in a supportive, collaborative environment.

For children with executive functioning deficits, a common challenge associated with ADHD, autism, and other cognitive disorders, cognitive-behavioral interventions often focus on improving skills related to planning, organization, time management, and self-regulation. Executive functioning skills are critical for academic success, as they enable children to set goals, prioritize tasks, and monitor their progress. Therapists and educators use cognitive-behavioral techniques to teach children how to develop routines, use checklists, break tasks into smaller parts, and monitor their own work. These strategies help children become more independent and effective learners, even when they face cognitive challenges.

Another cognitive-behavioral strategy that can be effective for children with learning delays is self-monitoring. Self-monitoring involves teaching children to become aware of their own behavior and cognitive processes, allowing them to make adjustments as needed. For example, a child might use a checklist to track whether they are staying on task during homework time or set goals for completing assignments within a certain time frame. Self-monitoring empowers children to take responsibility for their own learning and behavior, promoting a sense of control and accountability.

Parents and caregivers can also play an active role in cognitive-behavioral interventions by reinforcing positive thinking and behavior at home. For instance, parents might help their child practice relaxation techniques when they feel frustrated with a difficult task, or they might use praise and rewards to encourage perseverance and effort. By creating a consistent and supportive environment, both at home and in therapy, cognitive-behavioral interventions can help children with cognitive delays and learning challenges develop the skills they need to succeed.

Early Learning Strategies for Delayed Development

Early learning strategies are critical for addressing cognitive and learning delays during the most formative years of a child's life. Early intervention takes advantage of the brain's plasticity, or ability to change and adapt, particularly during the first few years of life when neural connections are rapidly forming. These strategies are designed to support the development of cognitive skills, such as attention, memory, language, and problem-solving, through age-appropriate, play-based activities.

One of the foundational principles of early learning interventions is scaffolding, a technique that involves providing children with the support they need to accomplish tasks slightly beyond their current abilities. The goal of scaffolding is to gradually reduce the level of assistance as the child gains confidence and mastery. For example, a parent or teacher might provide verbal prompts or physical guidance to help a child complete a puzzle, and over time, the child will learn to complete the puzzle independently. Scaffolding helps children build on their existing skills while encouraging them to take on new challenges.

For children with cognitive delays, language development is often a primary focus of early learning interventions. Children with delayed language skills may struggle with vocabulary, sentence structure, or comprehension, which can impact their ability to communicate and learn. Early learning programs, such as speech therapy or language-enrichment activities, provide targeted support for language development by engaging children in conversations, storytelling, and other interactive experiences that promote language use.

Parents and caregivers can support early language development by creating language-rich environments at home. This might involve reading books aloud, singing songs, playing word games, or simply talking with the child throughout the day. For example, narrating everyday activities, such as cooking dinner or getting dressed, helps children build their vocabulary and understand how language is used in different contexts. Repetition is key to language learning, so providing multiple opportunities for the child to hear and practice new words is essential.

For children with more significant cognitive delays, such as those associated with intellectual disabilities, early learning interventions often include structured play-based activities that promote cognitive development through exploration, imitation, and problem-solving. Activities like sorting objects by color or shape, building with blocks, or playing memory games help children develop important cognitive skills, such as categorization, spatial awareness, and working memory. Play is an especially powerful tool for cognitive development because it engages children in learning in a natural, enjoyable way.

Multi-sensory learning is another effective strategy for children with cognitive and learning delays. Multi-sensory approaches engage multiple senses—such as sight, sound, touch, and movement—during learning activities, which helps reinforce concepts and improve memory retention. For example, when teaching a child letters of the alphabet, a multi-sensory approach might involve tracing the letters in sand (touch), listening to the sound each letter makes (hearing), and watching a visual representation of the letter (sight). By engaging multiple senses, children with cognitive delays are more likely to retain the information and apply it to new situations.

Early learning interventions also emphasize the importance of routine and repetition. Children with cognitive delays often benefit from predictable routines, as they provide a sense of structure and security. For example, incorporating regular times for reading, playing, and practicing new skills helps children know what to expect and encourages consistent learning. Repetition is key in reinforcing cognitive skills, so practicing the same tasks or concepts multiple times can help children internalize and master new abilities.

Play-based learning remains central to early cognitive interventions. Encouraging imaginative play, cooperative games, and role-playing scenarios helps children develop problem-solving skills, creativity, and social cognition. For example, playing pretend in a kitchen set or a grocery store allows children to practice decision-making, sequencing, and language use in a social context. Play-based learning engages children in a fun, low-pressure environment while simultaneously promoting cognitive growth.

In addition to structured learning activities, sensory play—such as water play, sandboxes, or tactile exploration—can also help children with cognitive delays develop attention and sensory processing skills. Sensory play encourages exploration and curiosity, helping children make sense of the physical world and their place within it.

Tailoring Education Plans to Individual Needs

When it comes to addressing cognitive and learning delays, a one-size-fits-all approach rarely works. Each child has a unique profile of strengths and challenges, and their education plan must be tailored to meet their individual needs. Individualized Education Plans (IEPs) are a key tool for ensuring that children with cognitive delays receive the appropriate accommodations and support in school.

An Individualized Education Plan (IEP) is a legal document developed for children with disabilities who qualify for special education services. The IEP outlines the child's specific learning goals, the accommodations or modifications needed to support their learning, and the services they will receive (such as speech therapy, occupational therapy, or specialized instruction). The IEP is created in collaboration with a team that includes the child's parents, teachers, school administrators, and specialists, ensuring that the child's educational needs are fully understood and addressed.

The process of developing an IEP begins with a comprehensive evaluation to assess the child's cognitive, academic, and social-emotional functioning. This evaluation may include standardized tests, observations, and input from teachers and parents. Based on the results of the evaluation, the IEP team identifies specific areas where the child needs support and sets measurable goals to address these challenges. These goals are designed to be both realistic and ambitious, with the ultimate aim of helping the child progress academically and developmentally in line with their peers, to the extent possible.

Once the goals are established, the IEP outlines the specific accommodations and modifications that will be provided to support the child's learning. Accommodations refer to changes in how information is presented or how the child is allowed to demonstrate their learning. For example, a child with ADHD may receive extra time on tests or be allowed to take breaks during long tasks. A child with dyslexia might use audio books or have access to text-to-speech technology. These accommodations ensure that the child can access the curriculum without being hindered by their specific learning challenges.

Modifications, on the other hand, involve changes to what is being taught. For children with more significant cognitive delays, modifications might include simplifying the curriculum or breaking down complex tasks into smaller, more manageable steps. For example, a child with intellectual disabilities might be taught at a different grade level or be provided with alternative assignments that are more appropriate for their cognitive abilities. The goal of modifications is to ensure that the child is still learning and progressing, even if the content is tailored to their specific needs.

In addition to accommodations and modifications, the IEP also details the services and supports the child will receive. These may include specialized instruction from a special education teacher, speech or language therapy, occupational therapy, or behavioral support. The frequency and duration of these services are specified in the IEP, and progress is monitored regularly to ensure that the child is meeting their goals.

Regular progress reviews are an essential component of an IEP. The IEP team typically meets at least once a year to review the child's progress and make any necessary adjustments to the plan. If the child is making significant progress, the team may decide to increase the level of challenge in their academic work or reduce the amount of support they receive. Conversely, if the child is struggling to meet their goals, the team may decide to implement additional accommodations, modify the curriculum further, or increase the frequency of therapy sessions.

One of the most important aspects of tailoring education plans to individual needs is ensuring that the child is receiving a balanced approach to learning. This means not only focusing on academic skills but also addressing the child's social, emotional, and physical development. For children with cognitive delays, it is important to create opportunities for social interaction, as many of these children may struggle with forming relationships or engaging in social situations. The IEP might include goals for improving social skills, such as learning how to initiate conversations, take turns in games, or express emotions appropriately.

In some cases, children with cognitive delays benefit from inclusive education, where they are placed in a general education classroom with their typically developing peers. Inclusive education promotes social integration and allows children with cognitive delays to observe and learn from their peers. In inclusive settings, teachers often use differentiated instruction to meet the diverse needs of all students in the classroom. Differentiated instruction involves providing multiple ways for children to engage with the material, demonstrate their learning, and receive support. For example, a teacher might offer visual aids, hands-on activities, or group work to help children with different learning styles and abilities succeed.

For other children, a special education classroom or a hybrid model that combines time in both general and special education settings may be more appropriate. In these cases, the child may receive more intensive support in a smaller, specialized classroom environment for part of the day while participating in inclusive activities with their peers for the remainder. The IEP team works together to determine the best setting for the child based on their individual needs, strengths, and goals.

Parental involvement is a crucial element in the success of an IEP. Parents are encouraged to take an active role in the development and implementation of the plan by sharing their insights about their child's strengths, challenges, and progress. They are also vital advocates for their child's needs, ensuring that the IEP accurately reflects what will help the child succeed. Parents can work closely with teachers and therapists to reinforce strategies at home, monitor their child's progress, and ensure continuity between school and home environments.

Beyond the IEP, some children with cognitive and learning delays may also benefit from 504 plans, which provide accommodations under Section 504 of the Rehabilitation Act of 1973. A 504 plan is typically used for children who do not require special education services but still need specific accommodations to access the general education curriculum. For example, a child with ADHD might have a 504 plan that allows them to take tests in a quieter environment or receive extra time on assignments. Like IEPs, 504 plans are individualized and designed to meet the specific needs of the child, but they focus more on removing barriers to learning rather than modifying the curriculum.

Finally, for children with significant cognitive delays or intellectual disabilities, it is important to consider transition planning as they approach adolescence and young adulthood. Transition planning focuses on preparing the child for life after school, including higher education, employment, independent living, and community involvement. Transition plans are typically included in the IEP once the child reaches middle school or high school, and they are designed to ensure that the child is developing the skills they need to succeed in adulthood. This might involve teaching vocational skills, helping the child explore post-secondary education options, or working on life skills such as budgeting, cooking, or using public transportation.

Cognitive and learning interventions are essential for supporting children with developmental delays as they navigate the challenges of academic and social life. Through cognitive-behavioral interventions, early learning strategies, and individualized education plans, children can develop the cognitive, emotional, and social skills they need to succeed. These interventions provide not only the tools for learning but also the foundation for long-term growth, self-confidence, and independence.

By working closely with parents, educators, and therapists, children with cognitive and learning delays can receive the targeted support they need to overcome obstacles and achieve their full potential. Whether through structured early learning programs, tailored education plans, or cognitive-behavioral strategies, the goal is always the same: to empower children to thrive academically, socially, and personally, despite the challenges they may face.

Social and Emotional Interventions

S ocial and emotional development is a crucial aspect of a child's overall growth. It influences how children interact with their peers, manage their emotions, and form relationships with the people around them. When developmental delays affect a child's ability to understand social cues, regulate emotions, or navigate social interactions, targeted interventions become essential. These interventions help children develop the necessary skills to engage in meaningful social relationships, manage emotional challenges, and build self-confidence.

Children with social and emotional delays, such as those diagnosed with autism spectrum disorder (ASD), attention deficit hyperactivity disorder (ADHD), or other developmental and learning disabilities, often struggle with social interactions and emotional regulation. These challenges can lead to social isolation, frustration, anxiety, and difficulty functioning in group settings. However, with the right interventions, children can learn to manage their emotions, develop social skills, and participate more fully in their social worlds.

Social Skills Training for Children with Delays

One of the most important areas of intervention for children with social delays is social skills training. Social skills are necessary for interacting with others in a way that is respectful, effective, and appropriate. These skills include understanding social cues (such as body language or tone of voice), taking turns in conversation, sharing, cooperating with others, and handling conflicts. For children with developmental delays, these skills may not come naturally and often need to be explicitly taught through structured interventions.

Social skills training often begins with an assessment of the child's current social abilities and challenges. This assessment helps identify specific areas where the child may be struggling, such as initiating conversations, understanding non-verbal communication, or managing social anxiety. Based on this assessment, the therapist or educator develops a targeted intervention plan that addresses the child's unique needs.

Social skills training programs typically use role-playing, modeling, and direct instruction to teach children how to interact with others. For example, a therapist might model how to greet someone, ask for help, or join a group activity, and then have the child practice these skills in a controlled setting. Role-playing exercises allow the child to rehearse different social scenarios and receive feedback from the therapist on how to improve their responses. Over time, these rehearsals help the child gain confidence in their ability to navigate social interactions.

For children with autism, who often struggle with understanding non-verbal communication, social skills training might include exercises that focus on reading facial expressions and body language. Children may use picture cards or videos to practice identifying different emotions or social cues, and they can learn to apply this knowledge in real-life interactions. These exercises help children become more attuned to the emotions and intentions of others, which is a key component of effective communication.

Another important aspect of social skills training is teaching children how to manage social conflicts. Many children with social delays have difficulty navigating disagreements, resolving disputes, or negotiating with peers. Therapists use structured exercises to teach conflict resolution strategies, such as taking turns speaking, listening actively, and finding compromise. These skills are essential for maintaining healthy relationships and participating in group activities at school, home, or in the community.

Generalization of skills—the ability to apply learned social skills in a variety of contexts—is a critical goal of social skills training. Children often need support in transferring the skills they practice in therapy to real-world situations, such as interacting with peers at school, playing on the playground, or attending social events. Therapists and parents can work together to create opportunities for the child to practice social skills in everyday settings, gradually reducing the level of adult support as the child becomes more independent.

Parents and caregivers play a key role in reinforcing social skills outside of therapy. By providing regular opportunities for social interaction, such as play-dates or group activities, parents can help their child apply the skills they've learned in therapy. Parents are often encouraged to use social scripts at home—structured conversations or prompts that guide the child through specific social situations. For example, a social script might outline how to introduce oneself to a new friend, ask someone to play, or share toys. Over time, the child learns to use these scripts independently, improving their confidence in social settings.

Emotional Regulation Techniques

For children with emotional delays or challenges, learning how to regulate emotions is a key focus of intervention. Emotional regulation refers to the ability to manage and respond to emotional experiences in a healthy way. Children who struggle with emotional regulation may have difficulty controlling their reactions to stress, frustration, anger, or disappointment, which can lead to behavioral problems, social isolation, or emotional outbursts.

Emotional regulation techniques are designed to help children understand their emotions, recognize triggers, and develop strategies for managing strong feelings. These techniques are particularly important for children with ADHD, ASD, or anxiety disorders, as they often experience heightened emotions or difficulty processing and responding to emotional stimuli.

One of the most effective ways to teach emotional regulation is through cognitive-behavioral strategies that help children recognize and challenge unhelpful thoughts and behaviors. For example, a child who becomes easily frustrated when faced with a difficult task might learn to identify the negative thought patterns that contribute to their frustration ("I'll never be able to do this") and replace them with more positive, constructive thoughts ("I can try my best and ask for help if I need it"). By changing their thought processes, children can learn to approach challenges with a more positive mindset and manage their emotions more effectively.

Mindfulness and relaxation techniques are also widely used to help children regulate their emotions. Mindfulness involves paying attention to the present moment without judgment, which can help children become more aware of their emotions and how they are affecting their behavior. Simple mindfulness exercises, such as deep breathing, body scans, or guided imagery, can help children calm down when they feel overwhelmed or anxious. These techniques teach children to recognize physical signs of stress—such as a racing heart or tense muscles—and use relaxation strategies to regain control over their emotions.

For younger children, sensory-based strategies can be particularly helpful in managing emotional responses. Many children with developmental delays experience sensory sensitivities, which can contribute to emotional dysregulation. For example, a child might become overstimulated in a noisy or crowded environment, leading to feelings of anxiety or frustration. Occupational therapists often use sensory integration techniques to help children learn how to regulate their responses to sensory input. This might involve providing sensory breaks during the day, using weighted blankets, or engaging in calming activities like swinging, squeezing a stress ball, or listening to soft music.

Another key component of emotional regulation is teaching children how to label and express their emotions in appropriate ways. Many children with emotional delays have difficulty identifying their feelings or communicating them to others, which can lead to emotional outbursts or withdrawal. Therapists use emotion charts, feeling wheels, and other visual aids to help children learn to recognize different emotions and describe how they are feeling. For example, a child might use an emotion chart to point to a picture of a happy, sad, or angry face to indicate how they are feeling. Over time, the child learns to use words to describe their emotions, reducing the likelihood of behavioral problems caused by frustration or misunderstandings.

Parents can support emotional regulation at home by creating a calm-down corner or a designated space where the child can go to practice relaxation techniques when they are feeling overwhelmed. This space might include soft pillows, fidget toys, or sensory items that help the child calm down and regain control over their emotions. Encouraging the child to use this space when they need a break can help them develop self-regulation skills and learn to manage their emotions in a healthy way.

Emotional coaching is another strategy that parents can use to help their child learn emotional regulation. Emotional coaching involves acknowledging and validating the child's emotions while teaching them how to cope with difficult feelings. For example, if a child is upset because they lost a game, a parent might say, "I see that you're feeling frustrated because you didn't win. It's okay to feel frustrated, but let's take a few deep breaths and think about how we can handle it next time." By modeling healthy emotional responses and providing guidance, parents can help their child develop the tools they need to manage their emotions.

Group Therapy and Peer Interaction Support

Group therapy is a powerful intervention for children with social and emotional delays, as it provides opportunities for children to practice social skills and emotional regulation in a supportive, structured environment. In group therapy, children engage in guided activities with their peers, allowing them to learn from each other, build friendships, and develop important social and emotional skills.

One of the key benefits of group therapy is that it allows children to experience real-life social interactions in a controlled setting. For children who struggle with social anxiety, peer rejection, or difficulty understanding social cues, group therapy offers a safe space to practice interacting with others. Group leaders, often therapists or educators, facilitate activities that encourage cooperation, communication, and problem-solving, helping children apply the skills they have learned in individual therapy to group settings.

Social skills groups are a common form of group therapy for children with social delays. These groups focus on teaching children how to navigate social interactions, such as making friends, taking turns, and handling disagreements. Through structured activities like role-playing, group discussions, and cooperative games, children learn how to communicate effectively, share their thoughts and feelings, and resolve conflicts in a positive way. Social skills groups are especially beneficial for children with ASD or ADHD, as these children often need explicit instruction and practice in social interactions.

For children with emotional challenges, emotional regulation groups provide opportunities to practice coping skills in a group setting. These groups often focus on teaching children how to manage strong emotions, such as anger or anxiety, through techniques like deep breathing, progressive muscle relaxation, or cognitive restructuring. Group therapy allows children to observe how their peers cope with difficult emotions and learn from their experiences. The group setting also provides a sense of camaraderie and support, helping children feel less isolated in their struggles with emotional regulation.

In addition to practicing emotional regulation techniques, group therapy offers a platform for peer support and validation. Children who participate in group therapy often find comfort in realizing that they are not alone in their experiences. Sharing stories, listening to others, and providing mutual support fosters a sense of belonging and helps children build confidence in their ability to handle social and emotional challenges. This supportive environment is especially important for children who may feel isolated due to their developmental delays, as it encourages the development of friendships and positive social connections.

Play-based group therapy is another effective approach, particularly for younger children. In play-based groups, children engage in structured play activities that are designed to promote social interaction, cooperation, and emotional expression. For example, children might work together to build a block tower, play a group game, or engage in pretend play scenarios. These activities provide natural opportunities for children to practice taking turns, communicating with peers, and solving problems together. The group leader provides guidance and feedback as needed, helping children navigate any challenges that arise during play and encouraging positive social interactions.

For older children and adolescents, peer mentoring programs can be an effective way to provide social and emotional support. In peer mentoring, children with social or emotional challenges are paired with a peer who serves as a role model and provides guidance in navigating social situations. Peer mentors can offer valuable insights and support, helping children develop confidence in their social skills while fostering meaningful relationships. This type of intervention not only benefits the child receiving support but also provides leadership opportunities for the mentor, who gains experience in empathy, communication, and problem-solving.

Group activities in educational settings, such as circle time or group projects, are also opportunities for children to practice social and emotional skills in a less formal therapeutic setting. Teachers can facilitate group discussions on topics like emotions, friendships, or problem-solving, providing children with the chance to share their thoughts and learn from their peers. Group projects encourage cooperation and teamwork, while structured discussions help children practice active listening, empathy, and conflict resolution.

Family involvement in group therapy and peer interaction support is also essential. Parents and caregivers can attend family therapy sessions where they learn strategies to reinforce social and emotional skills at home. In these sessions, families can participate in role-playing exercises, discuss emotional regulation strategies, and explore ways to support their child's social development in daily life. Family therapy helps create consistency between the home and therapeutic environments, ensuring that children receive ongoing support in practicing the skills they've learned in group settings.

For children with more complex social and emotional needs, multidisciplinary approaches that combine individual therapy, group therapy, and peer interaction support may be necessary. These approaches involve collaboration between therapists, educators, and parents to create a comprehensive intervention plan that addresses the child's unique challenges. For example, a child with autism might receive individual social skills training with a therapist, participate in a social skills group at school, and engage in peer mentoring to practice interacting with classmates. This integrated approach ensures that the child is receiving support across different settings and contexts, promoting generalization of skills and long-term success.

Ultimately, the goal of social and emotional interventions is to help children develop the skills they need to form healthy relationships, manage their emotions, and thrive in social environments. Whether through structured social skills training, emotional regulation techniques, or group therapy, these interventions provide children with the tools to navigate the complexities of social interactions and emotional experiences. With the right support, children with social and emotional delays can build confidence in their abilities, develop meaningful connections with others, and achieve greater emotional well-being.

Sensory Processing Interventions

Sensory processing is the brain's ability to receive, interpret, and respond to sensory stimuli from the environment. For most individuals, this process happens automatically, allowing them to navigate and engage with their surroundings. However, for children with sensory processing disorders (SPD), this process can be disorganized or overstimulating, leading to significant challenges in daily functioning. Children with SPD may be hypersensitive (over-responsive) or hyposensitive (under-responsive) to stimuli, which can affect their ability to participate in everyday activities, regulate their emotions, and interact with others. Sensory processing issues are commonly seen in children with autism spectrum disorder (ASD), attention deficit hyperactivity disorder (ADHD), and developmental coordination disorder, but they can also occur independently.

Interventions that target sensory processing difficulties aim to help children better interpret and respond to sensory information. These interventions, often referred to as sensory integration therapy, are designed to provide structured sensory experiences that help the brain organize and process input more effectively. By supporting the child's ability to cope with sensory challenges, these interventions improve not only their sensory experiences but also their emotional regulation, social participation, and ability to focus and learn.

Understanding Sensory Processing Disorders

Sensory processing disorder is not a single diagnosis but rather an umbrella term used to describe a range of difficulties that occur when the brain has trouble receiving and responding to sensory input. Sensory processing issues can affect one or more of the sensory systems, including the senses of sight, sound, touch, taste, smell, balance (vestibular sense), and body awareness (proprioception).

Children with hypersensitivity (over-responsiveness) may find ordinary sensations overwhelming. For example, a child might cover their ears to block out everyday sounds, such as the noise of a vacuum cleaner or the chatter of a classroom. These children may be sensitive to bright lights, certain textures (like scratchy clothing), or even certain smells or tastes. As a result, they might avoid certain environments, foods, or activities, leading to difficulty engaging in school, social situations, or daily routines.

In contrast, children with hypo-sensitivity (under-responsiveness) may seek out sensory input, often in intense or risky ways. These children might not respond to sensations that others find uncomfortable or painful, such as extreme cold or heat. They may seek sensory stimulation by engaging in activities like excessive movement, crashing into furniture, or spinning. Hypo-sensitive children often crave more intense sensory input and may have difficulty sitting still or focusing because they are constantly trying to satisfy their need for stimulation.

In addition to hypersensitivity and hypo-sensitivity, some children experience sensory discrimination issues, where they have difficulty interpreting and distinguishing between different types of sensory input. For example, a child might struggle to judge the force needed to hold a pencil, leading to difficulty with writing. These children may also have poor coordination or difficulty understanding where their body is in space, making it hard to navigate their physical environment or engage in motor tasks like tying shoes or catching a ball.

Sensory processing disorders can have a profound impact on a child's emotional well-being, behavior, and ability to function in everyday life. Children with sensory challenges may become easily frustrated or overwhelmed, leading to emotional outbursts, anxiety, or withdrawal. In school, they may have difficulty concentrating, following directions, or engaging with peers, which can affect their academic and social development. At home, sensory issues can interfere with daily routines like eating, dressing, and bedtime.

Strategies for Sensory Integration

Sensory integration therapy is one of the most common interventions used to help children with sensory processing difficulties. Developed by occupational therapist Dr. A. Jean Ayres, sensory integration therapy is based on the idea that providing children with controlled sensory experiences can help their brains adapt and process sensory information more effectively. Sensory integration therapy is typically delivered by occupational therapists who are trained to work with children with sensory processing disorders.

The goal of sensory integration therapy is to help the child's brain become more organized and adaptive in its responses to sensory input. This is achieved through structured activities that expose the child to various sensory experiences in a controlled and playful manner. The therapist gradually increases the intensity and complexity of these activities, allowing the child to build tolerance to sensory stimuli and improve their sensory processing abilities.

Some common techniques used in sensory integration therapy include:

1. Vestibular Activities: The vestibular system, which helps control balance and spatial orientation, is often targeted in sensory integration therapy. Activities like swinging, spinning, and rocking help stimulate the vestibular system, promoting better balance and coordination. For children who are hypersensitive to vestibular input, gentle rocking or slow movement is often

introduced first, gradually progressing to more challenging activities as the child's tolerance increases.

2. Proprioceptive Activities: Proprioception refers to the sense of body awareness and the ability to perceive the position of one's limbs in space. Proprioceptive activities, such as jumping on a trampoline, lifting weights, or pushing heavy objects (e.g., a weighted cart or ball), provide deep pressure input that can be calming for children who seek sensory input. These activities also help improve body awareness, coordination, and motor planning.

3. Tactile Activities: For children with tactile defensiveness (hypersensitivity to touch), sensory integration therapy often includes exposure to different textures and sensations in a gradual, non-threatening way. Activities like playing with textured materials (e.g., sand, shaving cream, or water beads) or using sensory bins filled with rice, beans, or pasta help desensitize the child to tactile input and improve their ability to tolerate touch. For children with hypo-sensitivity to touch, these activities provide the necessary tactile stimulation that they crave.

4. Visual and Auditory Integration: Sensory integration therapy may also involve activities that help the child process visual and auditory stimuli more effectively. For example, children who are hypersensitive to light or sound may benefit from controlled exposure to bright lights, flashing objects, or varying levels of sound in a gradual and playful manner. Activities like tracking objects with the eyes, playing sound-based games, or using musical instruments can help children improve their ability to process visual and auditory information.

5. Sensory Diets: A sensory diet is a personalized plan of sensory activities designed to meet the specific needs of a child with sensory processing challenges. An occupational therapist creates the sensory diet based on the child's sensory preferences and sensitivities, incorporating activities that

provide the right balance of sensory input throughout the day. For example, a child who is hypo-sensitive to movement might have activities like jumping on a trampoline or riding a scooter scheduled throughout the day to help regulate their sensory needs, while a child who is hypersensitive to sound might use noise-canceling headphones during noisy times at school. Sensory diets are flexible and can be adjusted based on the child's changing needs and responses.

6. Deep Pressure and Weighted Tools: Many children with sensory processing issues benefit from deep pressure input, which can have a calming effect on the nervous system. Tools like weighted blankets, weighted vests, or compression garments provide constant, gentle pressure that helps regulate sensory input. Occupational therapists may also use massage techniques or brushing protocols to provide calming tactile input for children with tactile defensiveness.

Sensory-Friendly Environments at Home and School

Creating sensory-friendly environments at home and school is critical for helping children with sensory processing challenges feel more comfortable and successful in their daily activities. These environments are designed to reduce sensory overload while providing the appropriate amount of sensory input to meet the child's needs. By making small adjustments to the child's surroundings, parents, teachers, and caregivers can create spaces that support sensory integration and help the child regulate their responses to sensory stimuli.

At home, parents can implement several strategies to create a sensory-friendly environment:

1. Calm Spaces: Setting up a designated calm space or sensory corner where the child can retreat when they are feeling overwhelmed can be a helpful strategy for managing sensory overload. This space might include

soft lighting, calming music, and sensory tools like fidget toys, weighted blankets, or noise-canceling headphones. Providing the child with a quiet, safe space to relax and decompress helps them regain control over their emotions and sensory experiences.

2. Modifying Lighting and Sound: Children with sensory sensitivities to light and sound may benefit from adjustments in their home environment. Parents can use dimmable lights, blackout curtains, or lamps with soft, diffused lighting to reduce the intensity of visual stimuli. For children who are sensitive to sound, reducing background noise (such as turning off the TV or limiting loud conversations) or using white noise machines can help create a more soothing auditory environment.

3. Sensory Play Areas: Creating a sensory-rich play area at home allows children to engage in activities that meet their sensory needs. This might include a sandbox or water table for tactile play, a swing or mini-trampoline for vestibular input, or a variety of textures and materials for sensory exploration. Providing these sensory experiences in a controlled environment helps children regulate their sensory input and prevents sensory-seeking behaviors from becoming disruptive.

4. Structured Routines: Children with sensory processing issues often benefit from predictable routines, as they provide a sense of security and reduce the likelihood of sensory overload. Parents can establish consistent daily routines for activities like getting dressed, eating meals, or going to bed, incorporating sensory breaks as needed throughout the day. Sensory activities, such as brushing teeth with a specific type of toothbrush or wearing certain types of clothing, can be integrated into these routines to help the child manage their sensory needs.

At school, teachers and administrators can implement similar strategies to create sensory-friendly learning environments:

1. Flexible Seating Options: Providing flexible seating options, such as wobble stools, standing desks, or bean bags, allows children with sensory processing issues to find the most comfortable way to engage in learning. These seating options provide proprioceptive input and allow children to move or adjust their position as needed, helping them stay focused and regulated during classroom activities. For children who need more movement, fidget tools or sensory cushions can be provided to help them stay engaged without distracting others.

2. Quiet Zones: Similar to calm spaces at home, quiet zones in the classroom or school environment can provide a place for children to retreat when they are feeling overwhelmed by sensory input. These areas can be equipped with noise-canceling headphones, soft lighting, weighted blankets, or other calming tools that help the child decompress. Teachers can encourage children to use these quiet zones as needed, ensuring they have a safe space to regulate their sensory experiences during the school day.

3. Reducing Sensory Overload: In classrooms with children who are hyper-sensitive to sensory input, it is important to minimize sensory distractions. Teachers can reduce visual clutter by organizing materials and keeping classroom decorations minimal. For children with sound sensitivities, placing their desk in a quieter part of the room (away from doors, windows, or noisy equipment) or allowing them to wear noise-canceling headphones can help reduce auditory distractions.

4. Sensory Breaks: Incorporating scheduled sensory breaks throughout the school day can help children with sensory processing challenges stay focused and regulated. These breaks can include activities like jumping jacks, deep breathing exercises, or a short walk around the classroom. Providing these regular opportunities for movement and sensory input helps children manage their energy levels and focus on learning. For children with specific sensory needs, occupational therapists can work with teachers to develop a sensory diet that includes a variety of sensory activities tailored to the child's

individual needs.

5. Structured Transitions: Transitions between activities or locations can be difficult for children with sensory processing issues, as they may struggle with changes in sensory input or routines. Teachers can help by providing clear, structured transitions, such as using visual schedules, timers, or verbal cues to prepare the child for upcoming changes. Giving children extra time to transition between activities and allowing them to take sensory breaks during transitions can reduce anxiety and prevent sensory overload.

6. Sensory-Friendly Classrooms: For some children with significant sensory processing challenges, attending school in a traditional classroom setting may be overwhelming. Sensory-friendly classrooms are designed to provide a lower-stimulation environment where children can focus on learning without being overwhelmed by sensory input. These classrooms typically have fewer visual distractions, lower lighting, and quieter spaces, allowing children to engage in learning at their own pace. Teachers in sensory-friendly classrooms often use visual aids, calming routines, and sensory tools to support the child's learning and sensory needs.

Collaboration between occupational therapists, parents, and educators is essential for creating successful sensory-friendly environments at both home and school. Occupational therapists can assess the child's sensory needs and recommend specific strategies and tools that are tailored to their sensory profile. By working together, parents and educators can ensure that the child receives consistent support across different environments, helping them develop better sensory processing skills and improving their ability to participate in daily activities.

Individualized Sensory Plans can also be developed for children with more complex sensory processing challenges. These plans are similar to IEPs (Individualized Education Plans) but focus specifically on the child's sensory needs. An individualized sensory plan outlines the child's sensory preferences, triggers, and the accommodations or modifications that will be provided to help the child manage their sensory input. The plan may include details about sensory breaks, the use of sensory tools (like weighted blankets or noise-canceling headphones), and strategies for managing sensory overload during specific activities.

By creating sensory-friendly environments and providing targeted interventions, children with sensory processing disorders can learn to manage their sensory input more effectively, reducing the impact of sensory challenges on their daily lives. Sensory integration therapy, combined with accommodations at home and school, provides the tools and support these children need to thrive in both structured and unstructured settings.

Ultimately, understanding and addressing sensory processing challenges is key to helping children with sensory processing disorders achieve success in their social, academic, and emotional development. Through the use of sensory-friendly environments, individualized sensory plans, and collaborative support from caregivers and educators, children with sensory processing difficulties can experience greater comfort, self-regulation, and engagement in all aspects of their lives.

The Role of Parents and Caregivers

Parents and caregivers play a central role in the development and well-being of children, particularly for those with developmental delays or special needs. As the primary advocates, educators, and supporters of their children, they are key players in ensuring that their child's individual needs are met across different environments—at home, in school, and in healthcare settings. A strong partnership between parents, teachers, and healthcare providers is essential in building a support network that promotes the child's growth, learning, and emotional health.

This chapter will explore the vital responsibilities parents and caregivers hold in advocating for their child's needs, working collaboratively with professionals, and creating a nurturing and supportive home environment that fosters their child's development.

Advocating for Your Child's Needs

Advocating for a child with developmental delays or disabilities can be both empowering and challenging. Advocacy involves ensuring that the child's rights and needs are recognized and met by healthcare providers, educational institutions, and other support systems. Since children with developmental challenges may have difficulties expressing their needs or understanding complex situations, it is the role of parents and caregivers to be their voice and make sure they receive appropriate support and accommodations.

1. Understanding Your Child's Diagnosis and Needs

Effective advocacy starts with a clear understanding of the child's diagnosis, strengths, and challenges. When a child is first diagnosed with a developmental delay, disability, or learning disorder, it can be overwhelming for parents to navigate the complex information they receive from healthcare providers. Understanding the specific nature of the diagnosis—whether it involves cognitive, social, emotional, sensory, or motor delays—is essential for identifying the types of interventions and support the child may need.

Parents should take the time to learn about their child's condition, including common developmental patterns, potential challenges, and recommended treatments or therapies. Seeking information from trusted sources, such as healthcare providers, educational professionals, and reputable organizations (e.g., Autism Speaks, the National Down Syndrome Society), can help parents become well-informed advocates. Additionally, connecting with other parents who have children with similar diagnoses can provide valuable insights and support.

2. Advocating for Educational Accommodations

One of the most important areas where parents need to advocate for their child is within the educational system. Schools are legally required to provide appropriate services and accommodations to students with disabilities under laws such as the Individuals with Disabilities Education Act (IDEA) and Section 504 of the Rehabilitation Act. However, navigating these systems and ensuring that the child receives the appropriate services can be complex.

Parents play a critical role in ensuring that their child receives an Individualized Education Plan (IEP) or 504 Plan if they qualify for special education services. An IEP is a legal document that outlines the specific educational goals, accommodations, and services a child will receive in school. It is developed through a collaborative process between the child's parents, teachers, school administrators, and specialists. The IEP ensures that the child receives the necessary modifications and supports to succeed in the classroom.

To be effective advocates during the IEP process, parents should actively participate in IEP meetings, ask questions, and ensure that the plan is tailored to their child's unique needs. Parents should not hesitate to request additional evaluations or adjustments to the IEP if they feel their child's needs are not being fully addressed. Keeping detailed records of the child's progress and any concerns that arise can help parents advocate for adjustments to the plan over time.

In addition to securing an IEP or 504 Plan, parents can advocate for inclusive education where appropriate. Inclusive education involves placing children with developmental delays in general education classrooms alongside their typically developing peers, with the necessary accommodations and supports. This setting allows children to interact socially with peers, learn from a broader range of experiences, and participate in the general curriculum. Parents can advocate for inclusive practices by working closely with teachers and school administrators to ensure that their child has access to both academic and social opportunities in the school environment.

3. Advocating in Healthcare Settings

Healthcare advocacy is another essential responsibility for parents of children with developmental delays. Coordinating medical care, managing multiple appointments with specialists, and ensuring that the child receives appropriate therapeutic interventions (e.g., speech therapy, occupational therapy, physical therapy) require proactive communication and organization.

Parents should work closely with their child's pediatrician, developmental specialists, and therapists to ensure a comprehensive approach to care. This might involve advocating for additional testing, requesting referrals to specialists, or seeking second opinions if necessary. Understanding the treatment options available, asking for clear explanations of diagnoses and recommendations, and being involved in decision-making are all key aspects of effective healthcare advocacy.

Additionally, parents should ensure that healthcare providers understand the unique challenges their child faces. For example, a child with sensory sensitivities might need special accommodations during medical exams, such as a quieter environment or modified procedures to reduce anxiety. Advocating for these accommodations ensures that the child's experience in healthcare settings is as comfortable and supportive as possible.

Working with Teachers and Healthcare Providers

Collaboration between parents, teachers, and healthcare providers is critical for ensuring that children with developmental delays receive coordinated and consistent support. These professionals bring expertise and experience in their respective fields, while parents bring a deep understanding of their child's personality, needs, and preferences. When these parties work together, it creates a comprehensive support system that benefits the child in multiple areas of their life.

1. Building Collaborative Relationships with Teachers
   Teachers play a key role in a child's daily life and are often the first to notice any academic or social challenges a child may be facing in the classroom. Developing a strong partnership with teachers allows parents to stay informed about their child's progress and work together to address any difficulties that arise.

Parents can initiate open lines of communication with teachers by scheduling regular meetings or check-ins, where they discuss the child's progress and share insights into what strategies have been successful at home. Providing teachers with information about the child's specific needs—whether related to sensory processing, social interactions, or learning style—can help the teacher tailor their approach to support the child's development.

For example, if a child has difficulty staying focused in class due to ADHD, parents might share strategies that have worked at home, such as breaking tasks into smaller steps or using visual timers. Similarly, if a child has sensory sensitivities, parents might request accommodations such as seating the child in a quieter part of the classroom or allowing the child to use noise-canceling headphones during particularly loud activities.

Collaborating with teachers also involves reviewing and supporting the child's IEP or 504 Plan. Parents should ensure that the accommodations outlined in these plans are being implemented in the classroom and should discuss any concerns or successes with the teacher. If the child is making significant progress or facing new challenges, parents can work with the teacher and school team to adjust the plan as needed.

2. Collaborating with Healthcare Providers and Therapists

Just as parents collaborate with teachers, they also need to work closely with healthcare providers, including pediatricians, therapists, and specialists, to coordinate care for their child. This collaboration is especially important when a child receives multiple forms of therapy, such as speech therapy, occupational therapy, or physical therapy, as well as medical treatment for any related health conditions.

Parents should ensure that all members of the child's healthcare team are informed about the child's progress and any changes in behavior, health, or development. For example, if a child with sensory processing disorder starts a new therapy, it's important to share this information with the child's pediatrician so that they can monitor for any related effects or improvements.

It's also important to ask questions and clarify any recommendations made by healthcare providers. For example, if a therapist recommends a specific intervention, such as a sensory diet or a new approach to therapy, parents should feel comfortable asking how this intervention will benefit their child and what steps they can take at home to support it. Regular communication between parents and healthcare providers ensures that the child's treatment is consistent and that all interventions are aligned with the child's developmental goals.

3. Coordinating Care Across Settings

Children with developmental delays often require support in multiple settings—at home, in school, and in healthcare environments. To ensure that the child's care is coordinated, parents need to act as the central point of communication between all of the professionals involved in their child's care. This might involve sharing information between the child's teachers and therapists, providing healthcare providers with updates from the school, or coordinating meetings between the school team and healthcare professionals to discuss the child's progress.

For example, if a child's occupational therapist identifies a sensory issue that is affecting their ability to focus in school, the therapist can share this information with the teacher, who can then implement specific accommodations in the classroom. Similarly, if a child's IEP outlines goals related to speech development, the speech therapist should work closely with the teacher to ensure that these goals are being supported during classroom activities.

Creating a coordinated care plan that addresses the child's needs in all areas of their life helps ensure that they receive consistent support and are able to make progress across different settings.

Creating a Supportive Home Environment

While professional support in school and healthcare settings is crucial, the home environment plays an equally important role in the child's development. Parents and caregivers are responsible for creating a nurturing, structured, and supportive environment that promotes the child's growth, learning, and emotional well-being. This involves implementing strategies that address the child's unique needs, fostering positive relationships, and encouraging independence.

1. Establishing Routines and Structure

Children with developmental delays often benefit from predictable routines and clear structures at home. Routines provide a sense of stability and security, helping children know what to expect and reducing anxiety about transitions or changes. For example, having consistent routines for daily activities such as waking up, mealtimes, play, and bedtime can help children feel more comfortable and in control of their environment.

Parents can use visual schedules, timers, or checklists to help children understand the flow of the day and prepare for upcoming activities. For children who struggle with transitions, providing advance warnings or using visual timers can make it easier for them to shift from one activity to another. For example, if a child has difficulty moving from playtime to homework, parents can give a five-minute warning and show the child a timer so they can visually see how much time remains before the transition. Gradually, this structure can help the child become more adaptable and reduce the emotional stress that often accompanies unexpected changes.

In addition to daily routines, creating structured environments at home where learning and play are clearly defined can help children with developmental delays engage in meaningful activities. For example, setting up a dedicated homework space with limited distractions and organizing toys or materials in labeled bins can encourage independence and focus. Providing visual cues and consistency in how spaces are organized helps children understand what is expected of them in each area, whether it's for play, learning, or relaxation.

2. Encouraging Independence and Life Skills

Parents and caregivers can support their child's development by fostering independence and promoting the acquisition of life skills that will serve them in the future. While children with developmental delays may require more guidance in mastering certain tasks, giving them opportunities to practice independence is crucial for building confidence and self-efficacy.

For younger children, this may involve breaking tasks down into small, manageable steps and providing encouragement as they complete each step. For example, a child who struggles with dressing themselves might be taught to first put on socks and shoes, with more complex tasks like buttoning or zipping introduced gradually. Parents can use positive reinforcement, such as praise or small rewards, to motivate the child and celebrate their successes.

As children grow older, they can be given more responsibility for tasks like helping with household chores, managing a personal schedule, or preparing simple meals. Developing these life skills not only fosters independence but also helps children with developmental delays feel more capable and competent in handling everyday challenges.

3. Supporting Emotional and Social Development

Creating a supportive home environment also means addressing the child's emotional and social needs. Children with developmental delays may face difficulties in understanding or expressing their emotions, forming friendships, or navigating social situations. Parents play a crucial role in helping their child develop emotional intelligence and social skills.

Parents can support emotional development by modeling healthy emotional regulation and helping their child label and express their feelings. For example, if a child is frustrated because they can't complete a puzzle, parents can acknowledge the child's emotions by saying, "I see you're feeling frustrated because the puzzle is difficult. Let's take a break and try again." Teaching children to recognize and verbalize their emotions helps them manage frustration, anger, or sadness in a more constructive way.

In terms of social development, parents can provide opportunities for their child to practice social skills through play-dates, group activities, or family gatherings. For children who struggle with social interactions, parents can role-play social scenarios, such as introducing oneself or taking turns, to help the child practice these skills in a low-pressure setting before applying them in real-world situations.

4. Managing Sensory Needs at Home

For children with sensory processing disorders, creating a sensory-friendly home environment is key to helping them regulate their sensory experiences and reduce sensory overload. Parents can identify the specific sensory triggers that cause discomfort or distress for their child and make adjustments to the home environment to accommodate these needs.

For example, if a child is sensitive to noise, parents might use noise-canceling headphones or play calming music to create a quieter atmosphere. If a child seeks out sensory input, parents can provide tools like weighted blankets, sensory bins, or fidget toys to meet their child's sensory needs in a structured and safe way.

Establishing sensory breaks throughout the day can also be beneficial for children with sensory processing issues. Sensory breaks allow the child to engage in calming or stimulating activities, such as swinging, deep pressure exercises, or tactile play, that help them regulate their sensory input and maintain focus.

5. Promoting Positive Parent-Child Relationships

Above all, a supportive home environment is one in which the child feels loved, valued, and understood. Strong, positive relationships between parents and children form the foundation for healthy emotional development and create a sense of security that allows the child to thrive.

Parents can foster these relationships by spending quality time with their child, engaging in activities that the child enjoys, and showing empathy and patience during challenging moments. Open communication, where the child feels comfortable expressing their needs and emotions, helps build trust and strengthens the parent-child bond.

Parents should also be mindful of the need to care for their own emotional and mental well-being. Caring for a child with developmental delays can be demanding and stressful, and it's important for parents to seek support from friends, family, or support groups when needed. Taking time for self-care allows parents to maintain their energy and emotional resilience, which in turn benefits their relationship with their child.

Parents and caregivers hold an essential role in the lives of children with developmental delays, acting as advocates, collaborators, and providers of a supportive home environment. By advocating for their child's needs in educational and healthcare settings, building strong partnerships with professionals, and creating a nurturing space at home, parents can help their child reach their full potential. These efforts not only contribute to the child's cognitive, social, and emotional development but also lay the groundwork for a future where the child can grow into an independent and confident individual. Through ongoing collaboration and unwavering support, parents and caregivers empower their children to overcome challenges and succeed in all aspects of their lives.

Navigating School Systems and Special Education

The educational journey of a child with developmental delays or special needs is often shaped by a complex interplay of tailored support, accommodations, and collaborations between educators, parents, and healthcare professionals. Understanding how to navigate the school system and advocate for the appropriate educational setting for your child is crucial to their success. This chapter will delve into the details of the Individualized Education Plan (IEP) process, strategies for effective collaboration with educators, and the steps to finding the right educational setting for children with special needs.

The Individualized Education Plan (IEP) Process

The Individualized Education Plan (IEP) is a cornerstone of the special education process in the United States, mandated under the Individuals with Disabilities Education Act (IDEA). The purpose of the IEP is to create a tailored educational plan that addresses the specific needs of a child with disabilities and provides the necessary accommodations and services to help them succeed in school. Understanding the IEP process is critical for parents and caregivers, as it directly impacts the level of support and resources the child will receive.

1. Referral and Evaluation

The IEP process typically begins with a referral for evaluation. A referral can be made by a teacher, parent, or healthcare professional who has observed signs that a child may be struggling academically, socially, or behaviorally. Once a referral is made, the school will conduct a comprehensive evaluation to assess the child's needs. This evaluation may include academic testing, behavioral assessments, and input from specialists such as speech therapists, occupational therapists, or psychologists.

The evaluation process is designed to determine whether the child qualifies for special education services under IDEA and to identify the specific areas where support is needed. For example, a child with a learning disability may need accommodations related to reading or writing, while a child with autism spectrum disorder (ASD) may require social skills training or behavioral interventions. It is important for parents to be actively involved in this stage of the process by providing input, asking questions, and ensuring that the evaluation is thorough.

2. Developing the IEP

If the evaluation confirms that the child is eligible for special education services, the next step is to develop the IEP. The IEP is a formal document that outlines the child's current level of academic performance, their specific goals, the services they will receive, and the accommodations needed to help them access the curriculum. The IEP is developed by a team that includes the child's parents, teachers, school administrators, and specialists, such as speech or occupational therapists. This team approach ensures that the plan addresses all aspects of the child's needs.

During the IEP meeting, the team will set measurable goals for the child based on their individual needs. These goals are typically broken down into short-term objectives, which provide a road map for progress. For example, a goal might be to improve reading comprehension skills, with objectives that focus on increasing the child's ability to identify key details or summarize passages. The IEP also specifies the services and accommodations the child will receive, such as speech therapy, physical therapy, or one-on-one instructional support.

The IEP will also include accommodations and modifications to the general education curriculum. Accommodations are changes in how the child is taught or how they demonstrate what they have learned, such as providing extra time on tests, allowing for oral rather than written responses, or seating the child in a quieter part of the classroom. Modifications, on the other hand, involve changes to what the child is expected to learn. For instance, a child with intellectual disabilities may be working on a different academic level than their peers and require modified assignments that align with their cognitive abilities.

Parents are encouraged to actively participate in the development of the IEP by sharing their insights about their child's strengths, challenges, and learning style. They should also ask questions and ensure that the goals set for their child are realistic and achievable. It is important to remember that the IEP is a living document that can be adjusted as the child's needs change, so ongoing communication with the school team is essential.

3. Implementing the IEP

Once the IEP is developed and agreed upon, it must be implemented by the school. This means that all teachers, support staff, and specialists working with the child are responsible for ensuring that the accommodations and services outlined in the IEP are provided consistently. For example, if the IEP specifies that the child will receive speech therapy twice a week, the school is required to provide this service as part of the child's educational plan.

Parents play a key role in monitoring the implementation of the IEP. Regular communication with the child's teacher and service providers can help ensure that the child is receiving the support they need. Parents should also keep track of their child's progress by reviewing progress reports, attending parent-teacher conferences, and requesting updates from the IEP team. If parents notice that the child is not making progress or if they feel that the IEP is not being implemented properly, they have the right to request a meeting to discuss their concerns and make any necessary adjustments.

4. Reviewing and Revising the IEP

The IEP must be reviewed at least once a year to assess the child's progress and determine whether any changes need to be made to the goals, services, or accommodations. However, parents or educators can request a meeting to review the IEP at any time if there are concerns about the child's progress or if new challenges arise. For example, if a child has met their academic goals but is struggling socially, the IEP team might decide to add social skills training or counseling services to the plan.

Revisions to the IEP should always be based on data and observations about the child's progress. The IEP team will look at whether the child is meeting their goals, how they are responding to interventions, and whether any additional supports are needed. Parents are key members of this process and should feel empowered to advocate for any changes they believe will benefit their child.

Collaborating with Educators

Effective collaboration between parents and educators is essential for ensuring that a child with special needs receives the support they need to thrive in school. When parents and teachers work together, they can create a positive and cohesive learning environment that supports the child's academic, social, and emotional development.

1. Establishing Open Communication

The foundation of any successful collaboration is open and transparent communication. Parents should establish regular lines of communication with their child's teachers, whether through emails, phone calls, or in-person meetings. Regular check-ins allow both parties to stay informed about the child's progress, address any concerns, and make adjustments to support strategies as needed.

Parents can also ask for feedback on classroom strategies and share insights into what works well at home. For example, if a parent has found that using visual schedules or sensory breaks helps their child focus, they can share this information with the teacher, who may be able to implement similar strategies in the classroom. Likewise, teachers can provide feedback on how the child is responding to specific accommodations or interventions, allowing parents to reinforce these strategies at home.

2. Working as a Team

The IEP process emphasizes the importance of teamwork, with parents and educators working together to create and implement a plan that meets the child's needs. Parents should view themselves as equal partners in this process and feel empowered to voice their opinions and advocate for their child.

In some cases, parents may need to work with multiple professionals, including special education teachers, general education teachers, school counselors, and therapists. Coordinating with all members of the child's support team ensures that everyone is aligned in their approach and that the child is receiving consistent support across different settings. Parents can facilitate this coordination by attending IEP meetings, scheduling regular check-ins with teachers and specialists, and staying informed about their child's progress.

3. Supporting Learning at Home

Collaboration between parents and educators doesn't stop at the classroom door. Parents can play an active role in supporting their child's learning at home by reinforcing the skills and concepts taught at school. This might involve practicing reading or math skills, reviewing homework assignments, or working on social skills through structured activities. For children who receive specialized services, such as speech therapy or occupational therapy, parents can ask therapists for home-based activities or exercises to practice outside of school.

Providing consistency between home and school helps the child internalize what they have learned and apply their skills in different contexts. Parents can also model positive attitudes toward learning by encouraging curiosity, celebrating progress, and fostering a growth mindset. When children see their parents and teachers working together as a team, it reinforces the message that everyone is committed to their success.

Finding the Right Educational Setting

Choosing the right educational setting is one of the most important decisions parents and caregivers can make for a child with developmental delays or special needs. The goal is to find an environment where the child can thrive academically, socially, and emotionally while receiving the necessary accommodations and services to support their growth.

1. General Education vs. Special Education Settings
    Children with developmental delays or disabilities may be placed in general education classrooms, special education classrooms, or a combination of both, depending on their individual needs. The decision about placement is typically made during the IEP process, with input from parents, teachers, and specialists.

In a general education setting, children with special needs are integrated into classrooms with their typically developing peers. This setting is often referred to as inclusive education, where the child participates in the general curriculum alongside their peers but receives accommodations and support as outlined in their IEP. Inclusion can be highly beneficial for children with developmental delays, as it promotes social interaction, exposure to the general curriculum, and opportunities for peer learning.

However, for some children, a special education classroom may be a more appropriate setting, particularly if they require a more structured environment or specialized instruction that is not available in a general education classroom. Special education classrooms are often designed to provide smaller class sizes, individualized instruction, and targeted support for students with more significant learning or behavioral needs. These classrooms may focus on teaching life skills, providing academic instruction at the child's level, or offering more intensive behavioral support. While some children spend their entire school day in a special education setting, others may move between general and special education classrooms depending on the subject or activity.

In some cases, a hybrid model or resource room approach may be used, where the child attends a general education classroom for part of the day and receives specialized instruction or support in a separate resource room for specific subjects or skills. This model allows the child to benefit from inclusion in a general education environment while still receiving the individualized attention they need for certain areas of learning. The IEP team carefully considers which combination of settings is best suited to the child's abilities and needs.

2. Private and Charter Schools

In addition to public schools, parents may consider private schools or charter schools that offer specialized programs for children with developmental delays or disabilities. Some private schools are specifically designed to support students with learning disabilities, autism, ADHD, or other special needs, offering smaller class sizes, tailored curricula, and more individualized attention than what may be available in a public school setting.

Private schools may offer programs that emphasize alternative learning approaches, such as Montessori or Waldorf, which might be beneficial for children who thrive in nontraditional learning environments. These schools often prioritize hands-on, experiential learning, which can be particularly engaging for children with developmental delays.

Charter schools, which are publicly funded but operate independently of traditional school districts, may also offer specialized programs or approaches that cater to children with special needs. Parents who are interested in private or charter schools should thoroughly research the school's programs, qualifications of staff, and approach to supporting students with developmental delays. It's important to ensure that the school is equipped to meet the child's needs and provide the necessary services and accommodations.

3. Homeschooling and Virtual Learning

For some families, homeschooling or virtual learning may be a viable alternative to traditional school settings. Homeschooling offers parents the flexibility to create a customized educational plan that meets their child's unique needs, learning style, and pace. This option can be particularly beneficial for children who struggle in traditional classrooms due to sensory sensitivities, anxiety, or the need for more individualized instruction.

Homeschooling allows parents to incorporate therapeutic activities, such as speech or occupational therapy, directly into the child's daily routine. It also provides the opportunity to create a structured, supportive learning environment that minimizes distractions and caters to the child's sensory or behavioral needs. Parents who choose homeschooling should work with professionals to develop an educational plan that addresses both academic and developmental goals.

Virtual learning—whether through online schools or district-offered remote programs—can also be an option for children with special needs, especially in cases where in-person attendance is challenging. Virtual programs often provide a flexible schedule and the ability to learn from home, which can reduce sensory overload or anxiety in some children. However, it's important for parents to assess whether virtual learning provides enough interaction, structure, and support for their child, as some children with developmental delays may struggle with the lack of face-to-face instruction and social interaction.

4. Evaluating Educational Options

When selecting an educational setting, parents should take the time to carefully evaluate all available options to ensure that the chosen environment is well-suited to their child's needs. Visiting schools, observing classrooms, and meeting with teachers and administrators can provide valuable insight into how the school supports students with special needs. Parents should ask specific questions about the school's approach to special education, the qualifications of staff, the availability of support services (e.g., speech therapy, behavioral support), and the school's track record in working with children with developmental delays.

It's also important for parents to consider the social and emotional aspects of the school environment. Children with developmental delays often benefit from environments that are not only academically supportive but also nurturing and inclusive. Ensuring that the child will feel accepted and understood by their peers and teachers is crucial for their overall well-being and success.

5. Transitioning Between Educational Settings

As children grow and their needs change, they may transition between different educational settings over the course of their academic journey. For example, a child who starts in a special education classroom may eventually move into a general education setting as they make progress, or vice versa. Transitions between schools (e.g., from elementary to middle school) can also be challenging for children with developmental delays, as they may involve changes in routines, environments, and expectations.

Parents can help ease these transitions by working closely with the IEP team to plan for the change and prepare the child for what to expect. For example, visiting the new school, meeting with teachers, and discussing the child's goals and needs in advance can help create a smooth transition. Parents should also ensure that the child's new teachers and support staff are fully informed about their IEP and any specific accommodations or strategies that have been successful in the past.

6. Advocacy for Change

Throughout a child's educational journey, parents may find themselves advocating for changes to their child's educational setting or support services. If parents feel that their child's current placement is not meeting their needs, they have the right to request an IEP meeting to discuss alternative options or adjustments to the plan. For example, if a child is struggling academically in a general education classroom despite receiving accommodations, parents may advocate for additional support or a change in placement to a special education classroom.

Parents should also be aware of their rights under IDEA and other laws that protect children with disabilities. If parents encounter resistance or feel that their child's rights are not being upheld, they can seek legal advocacy or support from organizations that specialize in special education law.

Navigating the school system and special education can be a challenging but critical part of ensuring that children with developmental delays receive the support they need to succeed. By understanding the IEP process, collaborating effectively with educators, and carefully selecting the right educational setting, parents can help their child thrive academically, socially, and emotionally. Advocating for the child's needs and building strong partnerships with teachers and professionals creates a foundation for long-term success in school and beyond. Parents play a vital role in guiding their child through the educational system and ensuring that they have access to the resources and accommodations that allow them to reach their full potential.

Community Resources and Support

Navigating life with a child who has developmental delays can be overwhelming for parents and caregivers. However, a wide range of community resources, national programs, support groups, and financial assistance programs can help ease the burden by providing guidance, support, and practical solutions. Accessing these resources can make a significant difference in how families cope with the challenges of developmental delays, from securing therapies and interventions to finding a community of people who understand their experiences. This chapter will explore the various local and national programs available, how to find and engage with support networks, and ways to obtain financial assistance and navigate insurance.

Local and National Programs for Developmental Delays

The support available for children with developmental delays often comes from both local and national programs designed to help families access services, therapies, and educational resources. These programs provide crucial early interventions that can improve a child's cognitive, social, and physical development. Many of these programs also offer guidance to parents on how to advocate for their child's needs in school and healthcare settings.

1. Early Intervention Programs (Birth to Age 3)
   For children diagnosed with developmental delays during their first three years of life, Early Intervention (EI) programs offer some of the most critical

support. These programs are typically administered through state and local government agencies and are designed to provide therapies and services to help children reach developmental milestones. EI programs include services such as speech therapy, occupational therapy, physical therapy, and developmental therapy. They also provide family education and support to help parents and caregivers promote their child's development at home.

To qualify for EI services, children must undergo an evaluation to determine their developmental needs. If they are found eligible, a team of specialists works with the family to develop an Individualized Family Service Plan (IFSP), which outlines the goals for the child and the services they will receive. This plan is reviewed regularly to ensure the child is making progress, and adjustments are made as needed.

Parents can contact their state's Early Intervention office or the local department of health or education to initiate the evaluation process. The services provided through EI are typically free or offered on a sliding scale based on family income, making it accessible to many families.

2. Special Education Programs (Ages 3 and Up)

Once a child turns three, they may transition from Early Intervention to the public school system's special education services, which are mandated under the Individuals with Disabilities Education Act (IDEA). Through IDEA, schools are required to provide free and appropriate public education to children with disabilities, which includes developing an Individualized Education Plan (IEP) for each child based on their specific needs.

Special education services can include speech therapy, occupational therapy, physical therapy, behavioral interventions, and academic support. The goal is to help the child succeed in school while addressing any developmental challenges that might affect their learning or social interactions. These services are typically provided at no cost to the family.

In addition to IEPs, schools may also offer 504 Plans, which provide accommodations for children with disabilities that do not necessarily require special education but still need support to access the general education curriculum. Parents should contact their child's school or district to request an evaluation for special education services or to discuss their child's eligibility for a 504 Plan.

3. National Programs and Organizations

In addition to local programs, many national organizations offer support and resources for families dealing with developmental delays. These organizations provide information on diagnosis, treatment options, and strategies for advocating for a child's needs in various settings. They also offer community outreach, awareness campaigns, and funding for research aimed at improving the lives of children with developmental delays.

Some well-known national organizations include:

- The National Association for the Education of Young Children (NAEYC): Provides resources on early childhood education and developmental milestones.
- Autism Speaks: Offers information and resources for families of children with autism spectrum disorder (ASD), including toolkits for navigating the diagnostic process, accessing therapies, and finding local support services.
- The Arc: Advocates for individuals with intellectual and developmental disabilities, offering resources for early intervention, education, employment, and independent living.
- The Centers for Disease Control and Prevention (CDC): Offers information on developmental milestones, screening tools, and resources for children with developmental disabilities.
- National Down Syndrome Society (NDSS): Provides resources, advocacy, and support for individuals with Down syndrome and their families, including information on healthcare, education, and social inclusion.

These organizations can help families stay informed about new developments in research, therapies, and policy changes affecting individuals with developmental delays.

4. State and Local Government Programs

Many states offer additional resources and programs specifically designed to support children with developmental delays. These might include Medicaid waiver programs that cover the cost of therapies and healthcare services, State Children's Health Insurance Program (CHIP) for families who do not qualify for Medicaid but need assistance with medical expenses, or early childhood education initiatives that provide access to inclusive preschool programs.

Local health departments, school districts, and regional developmental centers often have information on state-funded programs and can guide families through the application process. It's important for parents to explore the resources available in their specific state, as each state may have different eligibility requirements and services.

Finding Support Groups and Networks

Support groups and networks can be an invaluable resource for parents and caregivers of children with developmental delays. These groups provide emotional support, practical advice, and a sense of community for families navigating similar challenges. Being part of a support network can reduce feelings of isolation, offer opportunities to share experiences, and provide a platform for learning about new strategies or resources that can help children thrive.

1. In-Person Support Groups

Local support groups offer parents and caregivers the chance to meet face-to-face with others who are going through similar experiences. These groups often provide a safe space for sharing concerns, discussing treatment options, and celebrating successes. Meetings may be facilitated by professionals such as social workers or therapists, or they may be run by parents who have experience raising children with developmental delays.

To find local support groups, parents can start by contacting their child's healthcare providers, Early Intervention coordinators, or special education teachers, who may be aware of community resources. Many hospitals and developmental clinics also offer support groups for families dealing with specific conditions, such as autism or Down syndrome.

In-person support groups often offer additional benefits, such as workshops, guest speakers, or opportunities for children to socialize with their peers in a supportive environment. Some groups even organize play-dates, family outings, or respite care services for parents who need a break.

2. Online Support Communities

For parents who may not have access to local support groups or who prefer the flexibility of connecting with others online, online support communities provide a convenient and accessible alternative. These communities, often found on social media platforms or specialized forums, allow parents to ask questions, share stories, and seek advice from a wide range of people across the country or even internationally.

Online communities can be particularly beneficial for families who live in rural areas or who have children with rare conditions, as they provide access to a broader network of individuals facing similar challenges. These platforms also offer the advantage of 24/7 availability, allowing parents to connect whenever they need support.

However, it's important for parents to carefully vet the online communities they join to ensure that the information shared is accurate and that the group maintains a positive, supportive atmosphere. Trusted national organizations, such as Autism Speaks or The Arc, often host or endorse online support groups that are moderated by professionals or experienced advocates.

3. Parent-Led Advocacy and Support Networks

In addition to traditional support groups, many parents find empowerment through participating in parent-led advocacy groups. These groups not only provide emotional support but also work to raise awareness, advocate for policy changes, and promote inclusion and accessibility for individuals with developmental delays.

Parents who are passionate about advocating for their child's rights in education, healthcare, or public services may find a sense of purpose and community in these networks. Parent-led advocacy groups often collaborate with national organizations, participate in public awareness campaigns, and lobby for legislative changes that benefit children with special needs.

Joining an advocacy group allows parents to connect with others who are similarly committed to making a difference while also providing them with tools and resources to better advocate for their own child.

Financial Assistance and Navigating Insurance

Raising a child with developmental delays often involves significant financial costs, from medical appointments and therapies to specialized equipment and educational services. Fortunately, there are several options for financial assistance, and understanding how to navigate insurance can help reduce the financial burden on families.

1. Medicaid and Children's Health Insurance Program (CHIP)

For families with limited income, Medicaid offers comprehensive coverage for children with developmental delays, including access to therapies, medical care, and long-term services such as case management and home-based care. Many states offer Medicaid waiver programs specifically for children with disabilities, which provide additional services beyond what is typically covered under Medicaid. These waivers often cover costs related to in-home care, respite services, and assistive technology.

The Children's Health Insurance Program (CHIP) is another option for families who may not qualify for Medicaid but still need help covering healthcare costs. CHIP provides low-cost coverage for children and typically includes doctor visits, prescription medications, hospital care, and, in some cases, therapies for developmental delays.

Parents can apply for Medicaid or CHIP through their state's health department or healthcare marketplace. It's important to review the eligibility requirements, as they vary by state, and to explore any additional benefits that may be available through waiver programs.

2. Private Insurance Coverage

For families with private health insurance, understanding the specific benefits and limitations of their policy is essential for accessing the necessary services for their child. Many private insurance plans cover a portion of the cost for therapies such as speech therapy, occupational therapy, and behavioral interventions, but coverage can vary widely depending on the plan.

Parents should thoroughly review their insurance policy to understand which therapies, treatments, and services are covered, as well as any limits on the number of sessions or the types of providers they can see. It is also essential to understand whether the insurance plan requires preauthorization for certain services or referrals from primary care doctors.

One common challenge for parents is navigating insurance claims for specialized therapies, such as Applied Behavior Analysis (ABA) for children with autism. While many insurance plans now cover ABA therapy due to legislative changes in various states, parents may still encounter roadblocks with approvals, reimbursement, or understanding their full benefits. In these cases, it can be helpful to work with a medical billing advocate or case manager who can guide parents through the claims process and help resolve issues with denied claims.

Appealing Denied Claims

If an insurance claim is denied, parents have the right to appeal the decision. The appeals process typically involves submitting a letter of medical necessity from the child's healthcare provider, along with documentation that demonstrates why the requested service or therapy is critical for the child's developmental progress. The appeals process can be time-consuming, but persistence can often result in successful outcomes, particularly when parents provide clear, evidence-based reasons for the requested coverage.

Parents should also keep thorough records of all correspondence with the insurance company, including phone calls, emails, and letters, to document their attempts to resolve the issue.

3. Supplemental Security Income (SSI) and Other Government Assistance

Children with severe disabilities may qualify for Supplemental Security Income (SSI), a federal program that provides monthly financial assistance to help cover the cost of medical care, therapies, and basic living expenses. To qualify for SSI, the child must meet specific medical and financial criteria, and the family's income must fall below a certain threshold.

In addition to SSI, some families may qualify for Temporary Assistance for Needy Families (TANF), a program that provides financial assistance and support services to low-income families. TANF can help cover essential expenses such as food, housing, and utilities, as well as provide access to job training and employment services for parents.

4. Grants and Non-Profit Financial Assistance Programs

Numerous non-profit organizations and foundations offer grants and financial assistance to families of children with developmental delays. These grants may cover the cost of therapies, medical treatments, assistive technology, or adaptive equipment. Some organizations also offer scholarships for special education programs, camps, or respite care for families who need temporary relief from care giving responsibilities.

A few notable organizations that provide financial assistance include:

- United-healthcare Children's Foundation: Offers medical grants to help cover health-related services not covered by insurance, such as therapies or assistive devices.
    - The Masonic Charity Foundation: Provides financial support for medical services, therapies, or special equipment for children with disabilities.
    - First Hand Foundation: Offers funding for healthcare, medical equipment, and therapy services for children with special needs.
    - Different Need Foundation: Provides financial assistance for children with developmental delays and their families to help cover the cost of therapies, medical equipment, and other needs.

Parents can search for financial assistance programs through national organizations, non-profits, or local community groups that specialize in supporting children with special needs.

5. Tax Credits and Deductions for Families with Special Needs
    Parents of children with developmental delays may also qualify for certain tax credits and deductions that can help offset the cost of medical expenses. For example, families may be eligible for the Dependent Care Credit, which helps cover the cost of care for a dependent child while the parents work or look for work.

In addition, families may be able to deduct out-of-pocket medical expenses related to their child's disability, including the cost of therapies, medications, medical equipment, and travel expenses to and from medical appointments, provided that these expenses exceed a certain percentage of their adjusted gross income.

Parents should consult with a tax professional to ensure that they are taking full advantage of the available credits and deductions.

Navigating Insurance and Financial Resources

Navigating the financial and insurance landscape can be one of the most daunting aspects of raising a child with developmental delays, but understanding the resources available can make it more manageable.

Working with Case Managers and Social Workers

Many families find it helpful to work with case managers or social workers who are knowledgeable about the resources and programs available to families of children with developmental delays. These professionals can assist with completing applications for Medicaid, SSI, or other government assistance programs. They can also help families find local non-profits that offer grants or services, advocate for the child's needs, and provide guidance on navigating complex systems, such as healthcare or special education.

Establishing a Special Needs Trust

For families who are concerned about long-term financial planning for a child with developmental delays, setting up a special needs trust may be a good option. A special needs trust is a legal arrangement that allows parents to set aside funds for their child's future care without jeopardizing the child's eligibility for government benefits such as Medicaid or SSI. The funds in the trust can be used to cover medical care, therapies, housing, and other needs throughout the child's life.

A financial planner who specializes in special needs can help families understand the benefits of establishing a trust and guide them through the process.

Community resources, support groups, and financial assistance programs are invaluable tools for families of children with developmental delays. From accessing local early intervention programs and school-based special education services to connecting with national organizations and online support communities, parents have a wide array of options to help their child thrive. By understanding the financial assistance programs available—such as Medicaid, SSI, and grants from non-profit organizations—parents can also alleviate some of the financial burdens associated with providing the necessary care and support for their child.

Navigating the complex world of insurance and financial aid may seem overwhelming, but with the right information, tools, and support, families can secure the services and assistance they need. By tapping into community resources and creating strong support networks, parents can find the guidance, emotional support, and financial help that will empower their child to succeed in every aspect of their life.

Long-Term Outlook and Transitioning to Adulthood

As children with developmental delays grow older, their needs evolve, and families face new challenges in preparing them for adulthood. This transition often involves developing independent living skills, planning for future employment or vocational opportunities, and addressing legal and financial concerns to ensure long-term care and security. With the right support, individuals with developmental delays can lead fulfilling lives, achieve independence to the extent possible, and make meaningful contributions to their communities. This chapter provides a comprehensive exploration of the key considerations and strategies for preparing children with developmental delays for adulthood, with a focus on independent living, vocational skills, legal planning, and success stories of individuals who have thrived despite the challenges they faced.

Preparing for the Future: Independent Living and Vocational Skills

One of the primary goals for parents of children with developmental delays is helping their child develop the skills needed to live as independently as possible. This process begins long before the child reaches adulthood, with a focus on building self-sufficiency, decision-making skills, and practical abilities. For some individuals, full independence may be achievable, while others may require supported or assisted living arrangements. Regardless of the level of independence, it's essential to provide opportunities for growth, skill-building, and community integration.

1. Developing Life Skills

The first step in preparing for independent living is teaching life skills that are necessary for daily functioning. These skills include personal care, household management, money handling, transportation, and meal preparation. For individuals with developmental delays, mastering these skills can take more time and may require structured teaching methods, repetition, and ongoing practice.

Parents can begin fostering life skills in childhood by assigning age-appropriate responsibilities, such as helping with chores, managing small amounts of money, or participating in meal preparation. As the child grows older, these tasks can gradually increase in complexity, leading to more independent tasks, such as doing laundry, grocery shopping, or managing a budget.

For individuals with intellectual disabilities or other cognitive challenges, breaking tasks down into smaller steps and using visual aids, checklists, or adaptive tools can help them better understand and complete daily tasks. For example, using a visual schedule for a morning routine or a step-by-step checklist for cooking a meal can provide the necessary structure to promote independence.

Life skills training can also be supported through transition programs offered by schools, local community centers, or vocational rehabilitation services. These programs often provide hands-on training in real-world settings, allowing individuals to practice their skills in a safe and supportive environment. Some programs also offer peer mentoring or job coaching to help individuals with developmental delays navigate the challenges of daily living and develop social connections.

2. Employment and Vocational Training

Vocational skills are another critical aspect of preparing individuals with developmental delays for adulthood. Meaningful employment not only provides financial independence but also fosters a sense of purpose, self-worth, and community involvement. While individuals with developmental delays may face barriers to employment, many can succeed in the workforce with the right training, accommodations, and support.

Vocational rehabilitation services are available in most states and are designed to help individuals with disabilities access job training, job placement, and employment support. These services typically begin during high school through transition planning, which is part of the Individualized Education Plan (IEP) process. Transition planning helps identify the student's interests, strengths, and career goals, and it outlines the steps needed to achieve those goals. For example, a student may participate in a work-study program, gain on-the-job experience through internships, or receive training in specific job-related skills.

Some individuals with developmental delays may benefit from supported employment, which provides ongoing assistance from a job coach or employment specialist. Supported employment programs match individuals with jobs that align with their abilities and interests, and they offer guidance in areas such as communication, task management, and social interactions in the workplace. These programs also work with employers to ensure that appropriate accommodations are in place, such as modified work tasks or flexible schedules.

In addition to traditional employment, many individuals with developmental delays find success in self-employment or entrepreneurship. This option allows for greater flexibility and autonomy, enabling individuals to work at their own pace and pursue their passions. Vocational programs can help individuals develop the skills needed to start and manage their own businesses, whether it's selling handmade crafts, offering freelance services, or running a small shop.

3. Supported Living Arrangements

For some individuals with developmental delays, independent living may not be fully achievable without ongoing support. In these cases, supported living arrangements offer a safe and structured environment where individuals can live semi-independently while receiving assistance with daily tasks, healthcare, and social activities. Supported living options range from group homes to assisted living facilities, where residents have varying degrees of autonomy based on their needs.

In a group home setting, individuals live with others who have similar support needs, and they receive help from trained staff with tasks such as meal preparation, medication management, and transportation. Group homes often emphasize community integration, encouraging residents to participate in social and recreational activities, both within the home and in the broader community.

Another option is assisted living, which provides more comprehensive support for individuals with significant medical or personal care needs. Assisted living facilities offer 24-hour supervision and access to healthcare services, while still promoting independence to the extent possible. These facilities are often more appropriate for individuals with physical disabilities, complex medical conditions, or cognitive impairments that require ongoing care.

For individuals who are able to live more independently but still need occasional support, independent living communities or shared living arrangements may be suitable. These communities offer housing with built-in support services, such as case management, social activities, and access to transportation. Residents in independent living communities may have their own apartments or homes but benefit from the shared resources and support available.

Legal Considerations: Guardianship and Financial Planning

As children with developmental delays transition into adulthood, legal considerations become increasingly important, particularly in terms of guardianship and financial planning. These legal decisions help ensure that individuals with disabilities have the appropriate level of support and protection as they navigate adulthood, while also securing their financial future.

1. Guardianship and Alternatives

When a child with developmental delays reaches the age of 18, they are legally considered an adult, even if they are not fully capable of making decisions independently. For some families, this raises concerns about the individual's ability to manage their healthcare, finances, and personal affairs. In these cases, parents or caregivers may seek guardianship to maintain the authority to make decisions on behalf of the individual.

Guardianship is a legal process in which a court appoints a guardian to act in the best interest of an adult who is unable to make decisions due to a disability or cognitive impairment. Guardianship can be full or limited, depending on the individual's level of functioning and needs. Full guardianship grants the guardian decision-making authority over all aspects of the individual's life, including healthcare, finances, education, and living arrangements. Limited guardianship, on the other hand, allows the individual to retain some decision-making authority, while the guardian oversees specific areas, such as medical decisions or financial management.

While guardianship provides a high level of protection, it also restricts the individual's rights. As a result, families should carefully consider whether guardianship is necessary or whether less restrictive alternatives may be more appropriate. Alternatives to guardianship include:

- Power of Attorney (POA): This legal arrangement allows the individual to designate someone they trust (such as a parent or caregiver) to make decisions on their behalf in specific areas, such as healthcare or finances, without taking away their legal rights.

- Supported Decision-Making: Supported decision-making is an alternative model that empowers individuals with disabilities to make their own decisions with the help of a trusted advisor or support network. This approach allows individuals to retain their autonomy while receiving guidance and support in areas where they may need help.

- Conservator ship: In some cases, a conservator ship may be established to manage the individual's financial affairs, without impacting their decision-making authority in other areas of life.

Families should consult with an attorney who specializes in disability law to determine the best legal arrangement for their situation and ensure that all necessary paperwork is in place before the individual reaches adulthood.

2. Financial Planning for the Future

Planning for the long-term financial security of a child with developmental delays is a critical aspect of transitioning to adulthood. Families need to consider how their child's needs will be met in the future, particularly in terms of housing, healthcare, and ongoing support. Fortunately, there are several financial planning tools available to help parents ensure their child's future is secure without jeopardizing their eligibility for government benefits.

One of the most important financial planning tools is the Special Needs Trust (SNT). A Special Needs Trust is a legal arrangement that allows families to set aside money for the individual's care without disqualifying them from receiving benefits like Medicaid or Supplemental Security Income (SSI). The funds in the trust can be used to pay for a wide range of expenses, including medical care, therapies, housing, and recreational activities. The trust is managed by a trustee, who is responsible for distributing the funds in the individual's best interest.

In addition to a Special Needs Trust, families may also consider setting up an ABLE account, which is a tax-advantaged savings account specifically designed for individuals with disabilities. ABLE accounts allow individuals to save money for qualified disability-related expenses, such as healthcare, education, and housing, without affecting their eligibility for public benefits. ABLE accounts are an excellent option for individuals who have more limited financial needs but still want to save for future expenses.

Families should work with a financial planner or estate planning attorney who is experienced in special needs planning to ensure that their child's financial future is protected. These professionals can help families establish the appropriate legal structures, maximize government benefits, and plan for the transfer of assets in a way that ensures ongoing support for the individual with developmental delays.

3. Government Benefits and Long-Term Support

Many individuals with developmental delays are eligible for government benefits that provide financial assistance and access to healthcare, housing, and support services. These benefits can be crucial for ensuring long-term stability, especially for individuals who may not be able to fully support themselves financially.

Two key programs that provide financial support for individuals with disabilities are Supplemental Security Income (SSI) and Social Security Disability Insurance (SSDI). SSI is a needs-based program that provides monthly cash payments to individuals with disabilities who have limited income and resources. SSDI, on the other hand, is available to individuals who have a work history and have paid into the Social Security system but are unable to work due to a disability. Both programs provide important financial assistance, but eligibility requirements differ, so families should explore both options to determine which program is the best fit for their child.

In addition to financial support, individuals with disabilities may qualify for Medicaid or Medicare to help cover healthcare costs. Medicaid provides health coverage to individuals with low income and limited resources, and it often covers services such as long-term care, home health services, and therapies that may not be covered by private insurance. Medicare, which is typically available to individuals who qualify for SSDI, covers hospital stays, doctor visits, and prescription medications.

Families should work with a benefits specialist or social worker to navigate the application process for these programs and ensure that the individual receives all the benefits they are entitled to. It's also important to stay informed about any changes in eligibility criteria or program requirements, as these can impact the individual's access to services.

Success Stories: Thriving with Developmental Delays

While transitioning to adulthood with developmental delays can present challenges, many individuals are able to achieve success in various aspects of their lives through persistence, support, and the right resources. The following success stories highlight individuals who have thrived despite their developmental delays, illustrating that with the right guidance and opportunities, it is possible to overcome obstacles and lead a fulfilling life.

1. Employment Success

For many individuals with developmental delays, finding meaningful employment is a significant milestone that brings a sense of purpose and independence. One success story is that of Jonathan, a young man with autism who, with the help of a job coach through a vocational rehabilitation program, secured a position at a local bakery. Jonathan's job responsibilities included preparing ingredients, cleaning equipment, and packaging baked goods for sale. Through on-the-job support and regular communication with his supervisor, Jonathan was able to build his confidence, develop new skills, and become an integral part of the bakery's team.

Jonathan's success is a testament to the value of supported employment programs, which not only match individuals with jobs suited to their abilities but also provide the ongoing support necessary to ensure success in the workplace. By focusing on his strengths and receiving the appropriate accommodations, Jonathan was able to thrive in his role and gain greater independence.

2. Independent Living

Another inspiring story is that of Mia, a young woman with Down syndrome who transitioned from living with her parents to a shared living arrangement in an independent living community. With the help of a case manager and support staff, Mia learned essential life skills such as managing her finances, preparing meals, and using public transportation. Over time, Mia became more confident in her ability to live independently while still having access to support when needed.

Mia's journey demonstrates the importance of life skills training and supported living options for individuals with developmental delays who want to achieve greater autonomy. By gradually building her skills and accessing the necessary resources, Mia was able to take control of her life and live in a community that provided both independence and security.

3. Advocacy and Community Engagement

Some individuals with developmental delays find their voice through advocacy and community involvement. Elijah, a young man with cerebral palsy, became an advocate for disability rights after attending workshops and conferences organized by local disability advocacy groups. Through his involvement in these groups, Elijah developed a passion for speaking out about issues such as accessibility, inclusion, and employment opportunities for individuals with disabilities.

Elijah's advocacy work led him to participate in public speaking engagements, where he shared his personal experiences and educated others about the challenges faced by individuals with developmental delays. His work has had a lasting impact on his community, promoting greater awareness and inclusivity. Elijah's success as an advocate underscores the importance of empowering individuals with developmental delays to take an active role in their communities and make a difference in the lives of others.

4. Higher Education

While some individuals with developmental delays may face challenges in traditional academic settings, many have found success through higher education programs designed to accommodate their unique learning needs. Sophia, a young woman with an intellectual disability, enrolled in a college program that offered specialized support for students with disabilities. The program provided academic accommodations, such as extended time on exams and access to a learning support center, as well as opportunities for social engagement and career development.

Sophia successfully completed her coursework and graduated with a certificate in hospitality management. She later secured a job at a hotel, where she applied the skills she had learned in her program. Sophia's success in higher education and her subsequent career demonstrate that with the right support and accommodations, individuals with developmental delays can pursue academic and professional goals that align with their interests and abilities.

Transitioning to adulthood with developmental delays presents unique challenges, but it also offers opportunities for growth, independence, and success. By focusing on life skills development, vocational training, legal planning, and community integration, families can help their children navigate the complexities of adulthood and achieve their full potential. Through careful planning and the right support, individuals with developmental delays can lead fulfilling lives, whether through meaningful employment, independent living, or active participation in their communities.

The success stories of individuals who have thrived despite their developmental delays serve as powerful reminders that, with perseverance, guidance, and access to resources, the future is full of possibilities. Families play a critical role in supporting their child's journey to adulthood, and with the right tools and planning, they can ensure a bright and hopeful future for their loved one.

Conclusion

The early years of a child's life are critical for their development, and for children with developmental delays, early intervention can make a profound difference in their ability to achieve their full potential. Throughout this book, we have explored the various aspects of recognizing and addressing developmental delays, from understanding the signs and accessing the appropriate services to providing support at home and in school. As we conclude, it is important to emphasize the key role that early action, positivist, and a proactive approach can play in helping children with developmental delays overcome challenges and succeed in life.

The Power of Early Intervention

Early intervention is one of the most powerful tools available to families of children with developmental delays. Research consistently shows that the earlier developmental challenges are identified and addressed, the better the outcomes for the child. This is because the brain is most adaptable during the early years of life, and early intervention capitalizes on this period of heightened neuroplasticity to help children build the foundational skills they need for future learning, communication, socialization, and independence.

1. The Impact of Early Identification

The first step in harnessing the power of early intervention is recognizing the signs of developmental delays as early as possible. Parents, caregivers, and healthcare providers are in the best position to observe a child's developmental milestones and identify any areas of concern. By paying close attention to how a child is progressing in areas such as speech, motor skills, social interactions, and cognitive abilities, families can seek evaluations and services at the earliest sign of difficulty.

Timely identification allows families to access the appropriate supports before delays become more pronounced or lead to secondary challenges, such as behavioral issues or academic struggles. Whether through formal developmental screenings at pediatric visits or informal observations at home, early detection is key to ensuring that children receive the help they need during the most critical period of brain development.

2. The Benefits of Early Intervention Programs

Once developmental delays are identified, enrolling a child in an early intervention program can provide them with the specialized services and therapies needed to address their specific challenges. Early intervention programs, which are available for children from birth to age three, offer a range of services, including speech therapy, occupational therapy, physical therapy, and developmental therapy. These services are delivered by trained professionals who work closely with families to create individualized plans that target the child's unique needs.

The benefits of early intervention extend beyond improving developmental outcomes; they also strengthen the bond between parents and children by empowering families with the knowledge and tools to support their child's growth. Parents who participate in early intervention programs often report feeling more confident in their ability to nurture their child's development, and they gain valuable insights into how to create a supportive and stimulating environment at home.

Moreover, early intervention can have long-lasting effects on a child's future success. Children who receive early intervention services are more likely to enter preschool and kindergarten with the skills they need to thrive in social and academic settings. This early support helps lay the groundwork for continued progress throughout their school years and into adulthood.

3. Reducing the Need for Long-Term Interventions

   One of the most significant advantages of early intervention is its potential to reduce the need for more intensive services later in life. By addressing developmental delays at a young age, children are better equipped to catch up to their peers and develop the skills needed for success in school and everyday life. While some children may continue to need support as they grow older, early intervention can often prevent delays from becoming more severe, minimizing the impact on the child's overall development.

For example, a child with speech and language delays who receives early speech therapy may develop the communication skills necessary to engage with peers and succeed in the classroom, reducing the need for special education services in elementary school. Similarly, a child with motor skill delays who receives physical or occupational therapy early on may gain the coordination and strength needed to participate in physical activities and daily tasks with greater independence.

By investing in early intervention, families can set their children on a path toward greater independence, academic achievement, and social-emotional well-being, while potentially reducing the long-term costs associated with more intensive interventions later in life.

Staying Positive and Proactive

Parenting a child with developmental delays can be an emotional journey, filled with moments of uncertainty, concern, and frustration. However, it is also a journey that offers countless opportunities for growth, learning, and connection. Throughout this process, maintaining a positive and proactive mindset is essential for both the child's well-being and the family's overall experience.

1. Cultivating Positivist in the Face of Challenges

It is natural for parents to feel a range of emotions when their child is diagnosed with a developmental delay. Feelings of guilt, worry, or fear about the future are common, and it can be difficult to adjust to the reality that their child may need extra support. However, it is important for parents to recognize that a developmental delay is not a reflection of their child's potential or their abilities as caregivers. With the right interventions and support, children with developmental delays can lead fulfilling, happy lives, and they often exceed expectations in remarkable ways.

Parents can cultivate positivist by focusing on their child's strengths and celebrating every milestone, no matter how small. Instead of comparing their child to others, parents can take pride in their child's unique abilities and progress. Additionally, surrounding themselves with a supportive community of family, friends, and professionals can help parents stay motivated and optimistic as they navigate the challenges of raising a child with special needs.

Finding joy in the everyday moments—whether it's watching their child master a new skill, share a smile, or express themselves in a new way—helps parents stay grounded and focused on the positive aspects of their child's journey.

2. Being Proactive in Seeking Resources and Support

One of the most powerful actions parents can take is to be proactive in seeking resources, services, and information that will benefit their child. The earlier families begin to explore their options, the more equipped they will be to make informed decisions about their child's care. This proactive approach includes staying informed about new therapies, educational programs, and community resources that may enhance their child's development.

Parents can also take an active role in advocating for their child's needs in various settings, whether it's working with healthcare providers to ensure their child receives the appropriate evaluations and treatments, or collaborating with educators to create an effective Individualized Education Plan (IEP). Advocacy is an ongoing process, and parents who are well-informed and confident in their ability to speak up for their child are more likely to secure the services and accommodations their child requires.

Being proactive also means staying open to new ideas and approaches. Developmental science is constantly evolving, and new therapies, technologies, and strategies are being developed to support children with developmental delays. By staying curious and exploring innovative solutions, parents can help their child access the most effective and up-to-date interventions available.

3. Building a Strong Support Network

Raising a child with developmental delays can feel isolating at times, but it is important for families to remember that they are not alone. Building a strong support network of family, friends, professionals, and other parents who understand their experiences can provide invaluable emotional and practical support. Support groups, both in-person and online, offer a safe space for parents to share their challenges, seek advice, and celebrate their child's achievements.

Professional support, such as that provided by therapists, counselors, and case managers, can also help families navigate the complexities of early intervention, special education, and healthcare systems. These professionals can offer guidance on everything from accessing services to managing the emotional toll of care giving. By reaching out for help and accepting support, parents can reduce stress and ensure that their child receives the best possible care.

A strong support network not only benefits parents but also creates a positive and nurturing environment for the child. Children thrive when they feel surrounded by love, understanding, and encouragement, and a supportive community can help foster that sense of security and belonging.

Fostering Resilience in Children and Families

Children with developmental delays often face unique challenges as they grow, but with the right support, they can develop resilience and adaptability that will serve them throughout their lives. Resilience is the ability to overcome adversity and bounce back from difficult experiences, and it is a quality that can be nurtured in both children and their families.

1. Encouraging Problem-Solving and Self-Advocacy

As children with developmental delays grow older, it is important to encourage them to take an active role in their own development. This includes teaching them problem-solving skills, helping them understand their strengths and challenges, and empowering them to advocate for their own needs. When children learn how to navigate obstacles and seek solutions, they build confidence and resilience.

Parents can foster self-advocacy by involving their child in discussions about their goals, preferences, and accommodations. For example, as a child becomes more aware of their learning style, they can begin to communicate to teachers how they learn best and what types of support help them succeed. Teaching children to express their needs in a constructive way prepares them for greater independence as they transition into adolescence and adulthood.

2. Nurturing Emotional Resilience

For both children and parents, emotional resilience is key to navigating the ups and downs of life with developmental delays. Emotional resilience allows individuals to cope with stress, disappointment, and frustration in a healthy way. Parents can help their child develop emotional resilience by teaching coping strategies, such as deep breathing, mindfulness, and positive self-talk.

Creating an environment where it is safe for children to express their emotions, ask for help, and learn from setbacks fosters emotional resilience.

Parents can model this behavior by openly discussing their own emotions, demonstrating healthy coping mechanisms, and showing that it's okay to seek support when needed.

In , taking action early is the cornerstone of ensuring that children with developmental delays have the best possible chance for success. The power of early intervention cannot be overstated—by identifying developmental challenges early and providing timely support, families can change the trajectory of their child's life, enabling them to reach their full potential. Whether through early intervention programs, therapies, or educational services, the support provided during a child's formative years lays the foundation for their future development and success. By addressing developmental delays early, parents can help their children overcome obstacles, build essential skills, and cultivate resilience that will benefit them for years to come.

Staying Positive and Proactive

Remaining positive and proactive in the face of challenges is essential for both parents and children. By focusing on what can be done rather than what cannot, families can shift their mindset to one of empowerment and growth. Positivist doesn't mean ignoring the difficulties that come with developmental delays, but it does mean recognizing the progress that has been made, celebrating small victories, and staying hopeful about the future.

1. Celebrating Progress

Every child progresses at their own pace, and it's important to celebrate each achievement along the way, no matter how small. A child's first words, learning to tie their shoes, or making a new friend are all milestones that deserve recognition. Celebrating these moments reinforces the child's self-esteem and motivates them to continue working hard, while also giving parents the emotional boost needed to keep going.

Parents can create positive reinforcement systems that encourage their child's growth, such as reward charts or praise for completed tasks. By focusing on what the child can do rather than on what they struggle with, parents can foster a sense of achievement and pride that helps build confidence.

2. Seeking Out Opportunities

Staying proactive means continually seeking out new opportunities for growth, learning, and support. This might involve exploring new therapies, enrolling in educational programs, or seeking out extracurricular activities that help the child develop social, emotional, and cognitive skills. The world is constantly evolving, and with advances in technology and understanding of developmental science, there are always new tools and resources to explore.

Parents should stay informed about the latest research, therapies, and educational techniques available for children with developmental delays. By staying curious and being willing to try new approaches, families can ensure that they are providing their child with the most up-to-date and effective interventions possible.

3. Advocating for Change

One of the most powerful ways parents can stay proactive is by becoming advocates for their child's needs. This can mean working with educators to ensure that the child receives the appropriate accommodations in school, collaborating with healthcare providers to access necessary services, or even joining advocacy groups that work to raise awareness and promote policy changes that benefit individuals with developmental delays.

Advocacy is an ongoing process, and parents who are informed, persistent, and assertive are often able to secure the services and supports their child needs to succeed. By sharing their experiences, parents can also contribute to broader efforts to improve the systems that serve children with developmental delays, ensuring that future generations have even better access to resources and opportunities.

150

Fostering Long-Term Success

The ultimate goal of early intervention, proactive parenting, and advocacy is to set children with developmental delays on a path toward long-term success. While every child's journey will be unique, the common thread is the importance of laying a strong foundation during the early years. By fostering a growth mindset, promoting independence, and ensuring that the child has the resources they need, families can help their child thrive in school, work, and life.

1. Building Independence and Self-Advocacy

As children grow older, helping them develop independence and self-advocacy skills becomes increasingly important. While early intervention focuses on building foundational skills, the next step is empowering children to take control of their own development. This means teaching them how to advocate for their needs in educational, social, and work environments.

Children with developmental delays should be encouraged to make decisions, set goals, and solve problems with guidance from their parents and teachers. Over time, these experiences help them develop the confidence and self-awareness needed to navigate the challenges of adolescence and adulthood. Whether it's learning how to ask for help, manage their schedule, or pursue their interests, fostering independence is key to long-term success.

2. Promoting Lifelong Learning

Success isn't just about reaching a certain milestone or goal—it's about maintaining a commitment to lifelong learning. For children with developmental delays, learning doesn't stop at the end of formal schooling. Whether through job training programs, vocational skills development, or continuing education, individuals with developmental delays should be encouraged to keep growing and adapting throughout their lives.

Parents can instill a love of learning in their children by encouraging curiosity, providing opportunities for exploration, and supporting their interests. By teaching children that learning is an ongoing process, parents can help them develop the resilience and adaptability needed to face new challenges and seize new opportunities.

3. Building a Supportive Community

Success is rarely achieved in isolation. Throughout life, having a strong support network is essential for overcoming challenges and maintaining well-being. This is especially true for individuals with developmental delays, who may rely on the support of family, friends, mentors, and professionals to navigate different stages of life.

Parents play a key role in helping their children build a supportive community. This may involve connecting with local organizations, participating in social groups, or fostering relationships with educators, therapists, and healthcare providers who can offer guidance and encouragement. A strong community not only provides emotional support but also offers practical resources that can help individuals with developmental delays achieve their goals and lead fulfilling lives.

In , taking early action is the most effective way to ensure that children with developmental delays have the opportunity to thrive. The power of early intervention, combined with a proactive and positive approach, can change the trajectory of a child's life. By recognizing the signs of developmental delays, seeking out the appropriate services, and staying engaged in their child's growth, parents can provide the foundation for long-term success.

It's important for families to remember that every child is unique, and there is no one-size-fits-all solution for developmental delays. What matters most is that parents remain committed to their child's well-being, stay open to new possibilities, and create an environment where the child feels supported, valued, and empowered to achieve their potential.

By taking action early, parents can help their children overcome obstacles, build essential skills, and create a future filled with possibility and promise. With the right support and a strong sense of community, children with developmental delays can lead happy, productive, and fulfilling lives, demonstrating that no challenge is too great when approached with determination, love, and a proactive mindset.